Changing Habits

The Caregivers' Total Workout

Endorsements for *Changing Habits*

- *"Changing Habits* presents an innovative program for good health and happiness: Activity Alleviates Anxiety. Debbie Mandel will help you find the balance between giving and receiving to transform stress into strength." **—Deepak Chopra, M.D.**

- "Debbie Mandel is an important voice in the growingly more verdant wilderness. A calling toward the warm health of self-liberation for so many women striving to break past the tree-line of our feeling 'lost in the dark wood of the world.' She has in her own life walked the walk and now extends a strong hand to those who too are attempting to complete their birth and become all they can be." **—Stephen Levine,** *Gradual Awakening* **and** *Unattended Sorrow*

- "Debbie Mandel reminds us that there are other reasons to exercise than the ones you have heard about. Yes, regular activity can reduce your risks for and help protect you against a number of physical illnesses. But it can also help people, especially people whose task it is to care for others . . . combat ailments that can't be measured by a cholesterol test or an EKG. Things like depression, disillusionment, sadness; the inner crises that can be almost as, if not equally detrimental to our health. Exercise can help you in that part of your life, too, and this book will show you how." **—John Hanc,** *Newsday*

- "Debbie Mandel's innovative and timely *Changing Habits* can change your life. So what are you waiting for? Jump on the bandwagon and read this book." **—S. Loyola M. Curtin, Parish Minister, St. Rose of Lima**

- "If you are a stressed out caregiver—whether by profession or simply because you see that as your lot in life—reading *Changing Habits* will make you feel better. Following the author's sensible recommendations for movement and exercise, plus heeding the wisdom of the caregivers who lend their voices to this book, will show you the way to better health, peace of mind, and an optimistic view of the future." **—John Nowinski,** *6 Questions That Can Change Your Life.*

- *"Changing Habits* provides straightforward advice for those living a stressful existence, bolstering the importance of the mind-body-spirit connection." **—Melody T. McCloud, M.D., OB/GYN** *Blessed Health: The African-American Woman's Guide to Physical & Spiritual Well-being*

- "Finally—an exercise program that truly encompasses body, mind and spirit. Mandel draws inspiration from a multitude of cultures and faiths to bring the reader uplifting, all-encompassing information about health and fitness. She takes such a positive approach to health, you can't help but be moved to live a happier, more active lifestyle." **—Liz Neporent**

Changing Habits

The Caregivers' Total Workout

Debbie Mandel

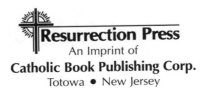

Resurrection Press
An Imprint of
Catholic Book Publishing Corp.
Totowa ● New Jersey

First published in September 2005 by Resurrection Press, Catholic Book Publishing Corp.

Copyright © 2005 by Debbie Mandel

ISBN 1-878718-98-3

Library of Congress Catalog Card Number: 2005927389

Cover design by Beth DeNapoli

Cover and inside photos by Michelle Kawka

Printed in the United States of America

1 2 3 4 5 6 7 8 9

Dedication

I simply want to say thank you to my friend and soul sister, Sister Peggy Tully, OP. The road is not difficult if you have a friend to take you by the hand.

Without Sr. Peggy's helpful suggestions, commitment and kindness this book would not have seen the light of day. She opened the door to a special community of women who spoke candidly, introspectively and humorously. Sister Peggy is an eloquent speaker and critical thinker. It is a joy to have a dialogue with her and it is serendipitous that we have crossed paths.

Acknowledgments

In loving memory of my mother Tuna Goldman Eisentadt who planted many seeds—all of them bloomed. I wrote *Changing Habits* in her honor.

A special loving thank you to my husband Steve who supported all my creative ventures—mind, body and spirit.

To my children, Michael, David, Amanda, my daughter-in-law Lisi and my cousin Esther Ettedgui for their sense of humor in putting up with my writing passion and high energy.

To Frank Mikulka whose fitness expertise, creativity and support helped shape *Changing Habits* and the Triple A Program.

To my literary agent, Linda Konner, who believed in the book from its conception and took me by the hand to guide me in the literary marketplace.

To Emilie Cerar for chiseling, sculpting and polishing *Changing Habits*.

To Michelle Kawka for her creative photographic vision and fine eye for detail.

To the participants of my stress-management groups who shared their stories with heartfelt emotion and honesty. My inner light greets your inner light.

Peace and blessings to all the Sisters who welcomed me, inspired me and trusted me. Your support has been invaluable.

Contents

Foreword

There are few things all doctors agree about, but one is the value of exercise. Exercise has so many beneficial effects that every specialty expounds the need for and the value of exercise. It benefits mood, brain, cardiac function and more. No organ suffers from sensible exercise and one's longevity is directly related to it. Every mile you walk adds time to your life.

The problem I see as I attend conferences is that people are more likely to bare their souls and deal with soulful problems than they are to expose their bodies and deal with their physical needs. Our bodies are a gift and without them we could not make a difference on the soulful or spiritual level because we would have no tools to work with.

So accept your body as a God-given gift and respect it and use it as your Creator intended.

Now I did not say to try and avoid dying by getting into excellent physical shape through exercise and eating a healthy diet and meditating regularly. Why do I say this? Because we all die and if you want to avoid psychotherapy in heaven then don't jog, meditate and eat vegetables to avoid dying. If you do you will be very bitter someday. The reason to do these things is to enhance the quality of your life and to bring you more joy and gratitude.

I exercise every day because I feel better doing it. But I don't feel guilty about not running a marathon every year if I do not want to put in the hours of training.

I ran my first marathon to help raise funds for cancer research. I spent many hours training and preparing myself for the marathon. I will never forget a woman standing on the sidewalk as I trotted by saying, "You're all winners." Life is a marathon, so live it to its fullest and you will be a winner too. It is not about the time it takes you to finish or the distance covered, but it is about the effort we put into every step along the way. At the end of the marathon every finisher receives a medal. It is not how fast you ran, but the fact that you finished what you started that you are rewarded for.

So read *Changing Habits* and start training for your life. After you complete the work outlined here make a list of the things it will take to make you the authentic human being you want to be. Now start practicing and training until you become the person you want to be. You are a winner, too. Look in the mirror and you will see the divine child and the gift you have been given: your body. If you find this hard to do, then treat yourself as well as you would your beloved pet. Take yourself for a walk and go on from there.

—BERNIE S. SIEGEL, MD
Author of *365 Prescriptions for the Soul*
and *Help Me to Heal*

Introduction

HOW IT ALL BEGAN

Nuns are the ultimate caregivers. The sisters have a lot to teach us through their inspiring and down-to-earth personal experiences. Traditionally, nuns have viewed their bodies as containers for the soul and dedicated their lives to service. And it is this distinct separation of mind and body as well as giving, giving and more giving that has led to stress and other health-related issues common to millions of women. Does all this sound familiar and resonate in your own life? The sisters have been receptive to changing their habits to break out of their traditional roles and to redefine their goals. If they can do it, so can you!

Changing Habits presents a comprehensive stress-management program which includes fitness and intelligent eating that I created for the Dominican Sisters of Queen of the Rosary in Amityville, New York where I was invited to bring the body into the equation of mind and spirit. This program offers strategies and concrete tools to every woman who lives sandwiched between her children and aging parents and to all women who are caught up in doing rather than being. Many have lost their personal identity—who they were before becoming a wife, mother and caretaker. *Changing Habits* is designed to create a healthy self-respect for body, mind and spirit.

Ironically, even though diet and fitness books line the bookstore shelves, Americans are more overweight and out of shape than ever before. While *Changing Habits* is not a cookie-cutter diet/fitness book, it helps the reader to take responsibility for her body, become fit and if necessary lose weight. It addresses the reality that we overeat, or eat the wrong things and fail to exercise because we ignore the root causes of poor health—stress and depression. It is the rare woman who doesn't eat to fill up an empty heart, who carves out enough time for exercise, or notices her energy levels dropping.

Changing Habits addresses the spiritual and fitness needs of all women who feel drained by their responsibilities, "good little girls" who are hungry for self-expression and soul-recognition. Because you may not know how or where to begin, I take you by the hand not only to explain exercises which can be done anywhere and without special equipment, but to go deep inside to address the heart and soul of movements that matter. What does it feel like *to mind that muscle*? Why am I afraid? What kind of benefits will I get from this? How much time is needed for this routine?

Although there are more than 44 million Americans, 18 and over, who provide some kind of voluntary in-home care for another adult or child (most likely both), the average age of caregivers is 46, and the majority are women. Women are brought up to be caregivers. *Changing Habits* will help you to see the whole context of your life and guide you to take a series of small actions leading to happiness. You will learn how to restore balance in order to take control of your life. Depression, anxiety, obesity, confusion, type 2 diabetes, cancer and arthritis do not have to be part of your aging process. Studies have shown that fitness and optimism can turn back the clock; exercise prevents, manages and cures many ailments.

Changing Habits is about giving birth to yourself many times over during the course of a lifetime. My mother taught me this in the way she lived her life with determination, honesty and compassion. I am my mother's daughter. Tuna Goldman, a holocaust survivor, came to this country with my father and an infant daughter, forging a fresh new life and learning the language of freedom and optimism. Although the three of us lived in poverty, we were not impoverished—we were rich in love and laughter. The view from our window was not pretty, but my mother transformed the landscape. Ignoring the planting directions on the back of seed packets, she scattered zinnia, salvia, marigold and morning glory seeds in shallow glass dishes and tea cups on our protruding window sill. My little girl eyes witnessed a miracle. All of the different flowers bloomed, a burst of color obscuring the dismal view. This is my legacy—a window sill garden.

My personal experience as a caregiver helped to shape *Changing Habits*. I have been a caregiver to two parents who had Alzheimer's disease, first my father and then my beloved mother. Since I was an only child, it all rested on my shoulders. While juggling terminally ill parents, a husband, three children and my work, I realized that I was just going through the motions without my usual sense of humor and cheerfulness. While some people feel fatigued and drained when they are mildly depressed, I rushed from one busy activity to the next to avoid thinking. There was an ache in my heart which wouldn't go away, but which somehow needed to be addressed.

Because writing is my passion, I felt intuitively that tapping my creativity would counteract my depression. I put this manuscript in my mother's hands like a beloved gift while she still had a glimmer of what it meant to both of us. And from this experience I learned that happiness means to be *reasonably happy* and that each one of us has the ability to experience happiness even in the midst of difficulty. This in fact, can make you appreciate and relish the good moments.

Changing Habits evolved easily and naturally from my first book, *Turn On Your Inner Light: Fitness for Body, Mind and Soul.* Having participated in my *Turn On Your Inner Light* stress-management workshop, Sister Peggy Tully, a Dominican Sister and friend, urged me to create a program for her community. For the first time convent life was demystified as I learned about the daily schedules of nuns and how much they could benefit from a strength-training program for body and spirit. Sister Peggy and I were ignited with creativity by our joint venture. I realized that it all hinged on having *strength in your faith and faith in your own strength.*

An inspiration can only go so far without a plan of action. I met with Sr. Peggy and the health director of the convent several times. I interviewed the sisters who were candid and embracing. Then I created a series of sessions, tweaking them as I went along to de-stress and strength-train nuns to help them live more fully with movements that would improve life quality. While I did not have to tell the nuns to *Turn On Their Inner Light,* I did have to tell them to turn it up a notch—to create a balance between giving and receiving and to make exercise and functional foods a part of their health regimen.

I consulted with Frank Mikulka, a trainer elite at the Hollywood Atrium Club in Lawrence, N.Y., a martial artist, boxing coach and former Marine about the fitness moves for the program. In fact, his exercises and fitness concepts were an integral part of *Turn On Your Inner Light*—the think-it and do-it outline for empowerment and happiness. Frank loved the idea of stress-management for nuns and how it would ripple down to all women. Flashing a smile, he said, "Since this originated with the nuns, let's call the program *Changing Habits.* I see this as a whole new movement!"

So whatever habits you have to change, this book will give you a jumpstart to move forward when you have lost the motivation to do what you know is good for you. You will learn the emotional tools to release the energy drains of resentment and unrealistic expectations to make room for a more *reasonable* happiness. When you feel unhappy and don't know why, just turn to the *Changing Habits'* Triple A Program for peace of mind, nourishing foods and functional fitness. *The difference between a sinner and a saint is that a saint keeps trying. Changing Habits* addresses the whole person—body, mind and spirit—so that you will soon feel happier, more self-confident and energized. So let's get started!

Chapter 1

THE TRIPLE A PROGRAM
ACTIVITY ALLEVIATES ANXIETY

ᢙᢩᠥᢆᠥ

We live in a fast-paced society filled with anxiety and stress. We can feel it in the air: terrorism, super germs and viruses, budget crises, and aging. No one is immune from anxiety—not even the sisters cloistered in the convent. Anxiety and sadness have a way of seeping into the cracks in the mortar of our homes and infiltrating the vents in the heating and cooling systems. Similarly, the sisters inhale the dark fumes of their community's concerns as well as their own families', just like any wife, mother and caretaker.

The Dominican Sisters of the Queen of the Rosary convent in Amityville, New York have learned from participating in the Changing Habits program that the quickest and healthiest way to shed stress is to move! If everyone would please rise from a seated or supine position and just move, then, within ten minutes we would all feel better. Don't take my word for it—just do it! Note: It takes 21 days to create a habit.

Why is exercise so important?

The following happens to your body when you exercise:

♦ **Stress hormones are shed.** Anxiety and worry drive up levels of cortisol, a hormone that interferes with digestion, regulation of the immune system, and other bodily processes—activating the instinctual preprogrammed fight-or-flight mode of behavior. If we are sitting on the couch or lying sleepless in bed while feeling anxious, we are not fighting or fleeing our demons. Instead we are caught in their grip. By interfering with bodily processes, cortisol literally eats away at us, chipping away at our bones. Note: osteoporosis has been linked to stress and depression. We need to decompress.

♦ **Endorphins are released.** Delicious feelings of well-being spread from the brain to the body. We begin to feel happier, lighter and more at ease. What bothered us just a few minutes ago, what seemed to have no solution, dissipates as we start to live in the moment.

♦ **We begin to think more clearly and increase our ability to focus.** Exercise drives oxygen into the brain and the muscles. Problems have solutions; obstacles are mere glitches when further analyzed. Instead of putting all our energy into worrying and complaining, we can now channel our energy into a solution.

♦ **We become empowered.** We begin to feel more confident and stronger. Our muscles and bones get stronger—if our skeletal frame is strengthened, the spirit is supported by a stronger *house*. The heart muscle beats more efficiently. The joints grow more flexible. As we work on our core balance and posture and stand straighter, the effect on the psyche is measurable.

♦ **We improve our health and prognosis rather quickly.** Changes are noticeable as soon as we become active. Those who suffer from metabolic syndrome, high blood pressure, type 2 diabetes, obesity, and high cholesterol levels would reap the greatest quantifiable benefits. This rapid change for the better improves the spirit because a sick body drags down the soul.

♦ **Exercise removes the fear of frailty that accompanies aging.** Many of us fear losing our independence and essential quality of life as we age. Exercise alleviates this worry because, unlike any genie in a bottle or external plastic surgery, exercise works from within to reverse the aging process. We become spry and stronger. Our minds grow sharper by learning new skills. We are less afraid of falling because we have built bone mass and improved our muscles.

♦ **We lower our risk of cancer.** Exercise has been shown to help prevent cancer by activating the immune system and shedding the stress that can serve as a trigger for cancer. How much easier to prevent than to cure! And should we develop cancer because of genetic or environmental triggers, the latest research shows that we may be able to walk our cancer away. Exercise boosts the effects of treatment and prolongs remission.

Being an empathic caregiver is an energy drain! Whether we are nuns or women in "the sandwich generation" taking care of parents and children, we can become depleted rather quickly if we do not take care of ourselves and maintain our balance. For example, Mary, thirty-eight years old, is the primary caregiver for her mother, husband, two sons, ages nine and eleven, a fourteen-year-old daughter, two cats, a dog, and fish. "I feel like everyone is lined up waiting for me all the time. Even the dog looks at me with big, hungry, brown eyes first thing in the morning. With all the animals in the house I feel like I live on a farm, working from dawn to dusk."

Mary wants everyone in her world to feel happy and protected. She tries to keep her whole family safe from mishap, pain and disappointment. She is an accomplished juggler. Not only does she run the house, but she works three-quarter time in a hectic pediatric office and is co-president of Family Ministry at her parish. She plans events for the church and is involved with the religious education of the children. However, Mary wishes that she could have a little more time to exercise to get rid of her stress. "I realize that exercise is healthy; I just don't make enough time for it because I am always doing for others. I'm the last one on my list. Good thing the dog needs to be walked, so I can accomplish two things at the same time. In good weather the dog and I do a brisk two-mile walk." If

Mary couldn't combine exercise with a task, she wouldn't find the time to do it. Sound familiar?

Because exercise is something we do for the self, it is the first activity to be cast aside with excuses like, "I don't have time," or "I'm just too worn out." The wonderful gift of exercise is that it organizes the day around good health. I am willing to bet that anyone who works out will also choose more wisely when eating and drinking, getting enough sleep and prioritizing daily problems. A person who exercises is more attuned to her body, sensing when something is amiss, such as a suspicious lump. She is able to take care of a physical ailment at the earliest warning signs when a disease is most responsive to cure.

Soul medicine: spirituality promotes good health

So what do you do when you are just plain overloaded? How do you find the time? Sometimes you have to clean out the clutter in your schedule; release what is no longer working or absolutely necessary. Sr. Peggy Tully shares her solution, "Until recently I was involved in a prison ministry that grew out of a course I taught at Molloy College. Part of that experience involved visiting the female prisoners at Riker's Island, Riverhead Jail and East Meadow Jail on Long Island. I would conduct prayer services for the female prisoners, distribute Holy Communion, and try to help the women find the still point within. Prisons are so noisy; there is no place to be quiet. I found the prison ministry meaningful for twenty-one years, but I needed to regroup and reset *myself*. I didn't have anyone to assist me, so I decided to let go of it. Hopefully some people have been helped. I am not the Messiah. I have to practice what I preach, which means taking care of my own needs, my body and my spirit."

Sr. Peggy's mission is to be contemplative and to give to others the fruits of that contemplation. She conveys the message that spirituality is holistic, not cut off from the experience of life. The goal is to become a complete person. "If I am depleted,

I cannot be spiritual and positive. In fact, if I really get run down, I could get sick. Spirituality does not exist only during prayer time; it runs through our lives. It is important for lay people to remember this in their active, busy lives."

Physical ailments link the body with the spirit and remind us of the mind's role in disease. Exercise activates and reminds us of that link in a healthy, positive way. When we are inordinately busy, concerned with being perfect and trying to accommodate our bosses, friends, family and co-workers, we may repress what we truly think and feel. We become so adept at subordinating our personal needs that we forget what we wanted for ourselves in the first place. We begin to feel the tension building at the disparity between our needs and what we think we must do. The next thing you know we are flat on our back—unable to "do" for anyone. When we are sick, a role reversal occurs: others take care of us. Now we have an excuse.

The severity of the illness often correlates to the degree of perfection we demand of ourselves and the level of control we need to exert in any situation. We set impossible standards for ourselves. We can't just be mothers; we have to be super moms. After all, we chose to stay home, so we had better be superior homemakers. Chronic Fatigue Syndrome usually afflicts high energy people (mostly women) who do things for everyone else, and do not sense their energy levels dropping. Suddenly, their energy reserves become depleted, and there is no safety net.

Enter Adrian, a woman in her late forties who regularly lifted weights in the gym where I work. She had lost her vitality, the sparkle in her eyes. Recently, I noticed that she was not frequenting the gym regularly. When I questioned her about these changes, she confided that she was suffering from fibromyalgia, which caused a burning sensation in the joints and interrupted her sleep. She went from doctor to doctor and was ultimately given a prescription for the antidepressant Paxil.

When Adrian described her symptoms to me, she claimed that she felt as though the blood was being drained from her arms. "Adrian, who is the blood relative draining your life?" I immediately asked.

"Oh my God, how did you know?" she responded.

I smiled, "I didn't know. You just told me." Right then and there Adrian realized that her illness was trying to tell her something. Although she had to take care of her twenty-something son, being a caregiver did not have to drive her life. Her son could take a back seat in her life.

When we develop a high tolerance for martyrdom, our bodies silently and secretly break down. Instead of waiting until we are sick before we can say, "No!" we have to learn to honor the immediate emotional signals the body emits.

As soon as we become aware of symptoms of stress like a backache, stomachache or headache, we need to stop what we are doing or thinking; we need to think objectively and shed the stress-damaging hormones. By reading where in the body our specific anxiety has lodged, interpreting the pain or discomfort, we can understand the underlying problem and begin to correct it. The body serves as a metaphor for the specific spiritual uneasiness. Why do we experience pain in a specific location? What does it mean spiritually?

- ♦ A pain in the upper back may mean that we shoulder too many responsibilities.
- ♦ A pain in the middle back implies that we feel unsupported.
- ♦ A stomachache may mean that our egos are on the line; that is why children get stomachaches during exams.
- ♦ Chest pain may mean grief.
- ♦ Joint pains imply the fear of moving forward.
- ♦ Skin eruptions are associated with our anger.
- ♦ Visual or auditory problems often indicate that you don't want to see or hear something.

See how easy it is. We can all become medical intuitives in the *university of life*—and without a medical degree.

It's time to open our eyes and see that many women's lives are shortened by giving away too much of themselves. In general, women absorb stress, are overworked, eat to fill up emotionally and forget to take care of themselves. Not a healthy lifestyle!

Sr. Helen of the Benedictine Order is in charge of the Wellness Program in Erie, Pennsylvania. Her job is to educate the church community about prevention of illness and disease. Personally, she has had a major breakthrough. "I have emerged from a life of spending-it-all-for-Jesus and He-will-take-care-of-us selflessness. Today I preach the notion that the self is important, that the self should be put first, so that you can launch into the activities of daily living pain free and energized, ever mindful of the wondrous mind-body relationship. This essentially is care for the caregiver. Isn't that what Jesus taught—care of the self, others, and the earth? Because of years of deprivation as a religious sister, I have trouble practicing what I preach. How ironic that taking care of my health is stressful and difficult!"

Following a health regimen is stressful for Sr. Helen since she feels it is like having another child to take care of. Her ministry comes first, then community life, followed by dealing with her complex personality; last on the list is a healthy lifestyle of diet and fitness. She finds it stressful to relieve stress! For example, she just finished a de-stressing assignment from her support group to send a valentine to herself. "Imagine fifty-nine years old and I'm valentining." Here's what she wrote, "So, Helen, you slipped for a month or so on your food and exercise plan. Next time remember to keep your larder stocked with no-fat items. Remember to cook your whole-wheat pasta, to go to the salad bar two times a day, eat your whole grains right along with the sugars that you are overdosing on and drink a bottle of water with the sweets. Make an emergency tape for yourself to listen to, one that encourages you, tries to reason with you while supporting yourself and above all do it all l-o-v-**I**-n-g-l-y, with great kindness for yourself, of course. When you can't comply with the nutrition modality of your program, try to do the other three components no matter what: stress management, exercise and group support. Picture a future of flexibility and energy for your days in this progressive and vital community, pain-free and delicious. I want this for you, dear Helen. The world needs this for you."

Sr. Helen recognizes that she is currently experiencing a tug of war between her health and her emotions because her upbringing in the church emphasized the mind while it negated the body, even suggesting that the body was bad or at best needed to be brought under control. "I know that is why I embrace the whole mind-body concept in wellness today. I feel that I have a deep well of grief that I dip into when any new, unsettling things happen. I believe that I have to work on my body to help heal the past."

Her baggage from childhood, like that of many women, is anger. As a girl she was raised to be seen and not heard. The anger also stems from a church that didn't have much of a place for girls when she was growing up. Her anger? It grew from a community that was devoted to the daily routine and the details. And now that she has come of age, it is a challenge for her to release the anger that has wreaked havoc with her cardiac health and diabetes. "No one's to blame for not flowering, but myself," she observes.

Exercise control over your life

Of course, we can all identify with Sr. Helen's problems and we can all do something about them. Here is how to move forward:

Look at exercise as your lifeline

By exercising we are exercising the right to make time for the self, get rid of toxic stress, release the happiness hormones and most importantly generate the life-giving force that is our birthright. As a selfless wife, mother or daughter of aging parents, you should think of it this way: When the oxygen mask drops down from the overhead cabin of an airplane, you are instructed to first put it on your face and then on the face of the child sitting next to you. If you pass out, your charge is unattended and helpless. Exercise is your lifeline, your oxygen mask. It will extend your life and give you greater function, even stimulate your brain. After all, it is not about how long you live, but how much life there is in your years.

The challenge is: how to get a stressed, over-scheduled person to exercise? This problem reminds me of the fairy tale *Snow White and the Seven Dwarfs*. One of the dwarfs, Grumpy, is unhappy and proclaims, "I don't want to be happy; I want to be sad!" Clinging to a stressed state gives a person something he or she is seeking—attention and concern—"Take care of me. I'm a victim." Sr. Diane Capuano, Vocation Director for the Dominican Sisters of Amityville, advises caregivers, not to get caught up in the dynamics of nurturing and nursing, letting it take over your whole identity. Everyone needs a variety of support systems. She realizes that sometimes we even feel guilty about having a good time. Think about the expression *I'm so happy, I can't stand it!* Language is emotionally revealing. It becomes difficult to negotiate our dependency and caregiving. We tend to forget that we have a right to live our own life and find happiness.

Realize that exercise empowers you

Exercise physically and mentally empowers the self, awakening the potential to grow and move on. For example, I have observed women who felt unsatisfied and uncomfortable in their job and marriage, or felt pressured to be the perfect mother or daughter. Then they began a strength-training program. After about a year they were able to change their own dynamics to find greater fulfillment. As they put on more muscle, coordinated their movements and improved their balance, they transferred these skills to their emotional lives. Training involves *core stability first, then mobility.* As they looked better and felt healthier, they blossomed with a new-found creative force and, most importantly, self-confidence. They continued to exercise regularly because of these motivating benefits, which gave them the ability to look at their "smaller" problems and see the total picture—then the solution. Practicing a daily regimen of exercise awakens the senses to greater pleasure in life.

Follow these simple guidelines when you are experiencing an energy crash due to bouts of intense busyness:

- Become aware of your feelings. Realize what depletes you and whether you are distracting yourself from confronting an issue.

- Notice how uncomfortable you are. This will motivate you to change and to make every effort to pull yourself out of it. Conceptualize exercise as deliberate *movements that matter,* not as something you hate to do. Exercise will help organize your day around good health.

- Make small changes gradually. As the saying goes, *small steps, giant gains.* Think of all the New Year's resolutions about getting fit that we don't keep. Instead, call them New Year's *evolutions,* and be patient. Progress is not a straight line. Compliment yourself frequently for keeping up the good work.

- Work out with a friend. Sometimes we need an angel to take us by the hand, a friend to serve as a positive mirror. Often we are sad because we feel lonely. Working out with a buddy becomes a social and positive experience. It cements a healthy bond—even without speaking. If you don't have a friend to exercise with, go to the gym. You will meet people and make friends; many people form close ties when they sweat together.

- Sign up for exercise classes in a gym or community center.

Try aerobics, spinning, interval training, body-sculpting, yoga, Pilates, and dancing. Just signing up for a class, like scheduling an appointment with a doctor, makes you feel better! Also, a class is more effective than a treadmill or stationary bicycle, as you need to tap into group energy. If you don't like classes and would rather work out in the privacy of your home, get a trainer for a few sessions to show you what to do, or get a video. The Changing Habits program in Chapter 13 demonstrates fun exercises you can do at home using your body's own resistance for head-to-toe fitness. The movements are designed to help you get stronger to tackle activities of daily life.

♦ Listen to music while exercising to create a synergistic effect, boosting mental acuity. The pulsating music works to excite and keep you moving.

♦ Put on your sneakers and walk out the door. Sunlight will energize you. A brisk walk will de-stress you. Aim for a twenty-minute walk, and each time try to pick up the pace a little more. To add excitement, walk briskly for five minutes, then slow down and walk at a relaxed pace for two minutes. Then pick up the pace for five minutes; next stroll for two minutes. Continue the cycle. Varying the intervals perks up the body and your mood, keeps you interested, alert and involved. When this routine becomes a habit, pump your arms and sprint for a one-minute interval. Before you know it, you may be jogging and experiencing a runner's high! The most advanced walkers can wear a weighted vest while walking to add a strength training component to the upper body as well as increase the intensity level.

♦ Buy a new pair of sneakers, fitness clothes, or a workout audio/video. These can help you to get into the exercise groove. Remember how anxious you felt before the first day of school? Your mother bought you some new clothes along with a new book bag, pencil case, lunch box. Well, you get the idea.

◆ Post motivating quotes (like the Self-Care mantras at the end of every chapter) all over your home, as a screen saver or on the refrigerator. Play motivating music—perhaps the theme song from *Rocky*.

◆ To keep motivation at an all-time high, change your routine every four to six weeks. Remember that nothing deadens the heart like routine. Your workout mirrors your life!

Try this: Exercise together with the people you take care of (if possible) or work with. The energy released will be healing for all of you. After you have worked out together for about ten or fifteen minutes, your sense of humor will be activated. Negotiation will be easier and more fruitful. That's why so many business and political deals are sealed on the golf course. Balance your energy while you balance those in your care. Sweat makes it all small stuff.

Life is a precious gift. We each have a mission to complete: to live an authentic, personally rewarding life. To be the best that we can be we need to generate feelings of happiness and serenity. If you are a caregiver, your anxiety and unhappiness are transmitted to those around you. Your happiness and calmness are also conveyed to others. Exercise will physiologically and spiritually restore your balance. Therefore it is your moral obligation to exercise to generate positive feelings which in turn transfer to others who will, in turn, pay it forward.

Self-care Mantras

◆ Practicing a daily regimen of exercise awakens the senses to greater pleasure.

◆ Exercise the right to make time for yourself.

◆ Small steps, giant gains.

◆ Nothing deadens the heart like routine.

◆ Sweat makes it all small stuff.

Chapter 2

TURN STRESS INTO STRENGTH

When I run a stress-reduction workshop, particularly for a new group, I see hopeful participants with anxious eyes, waiting for me to whip out my magic wand and make them stress-free and serene. Not only is this an unrealistic expectation, it isn't healthy either! The latest research shows that a little stress is good for you because it wakes up your senses and alerts the immune system to be vigilant.

Stress is part of life, whether you live in a big city or in a small town. The longer you live, the more stress you encounter. Media coverage brings it home daily in a sensational style. For example, last year's flu epidemic was over-dramatized. It took awhile for people to realize that the same photographs of children who had died were being shown repeatedly and did not represent new victims. Broadcasters followed up the news that American cows were infected with "madness" with announcements that farmed salmon was replete with cancer-causing PCBs. Suddenly, steak didn't seem all that unhealthy anymore.

For Joanne of Merrick, New York, a constant stressor is trying to be a good parent. "What I had to do over the years was to make peace with the concept that some days I'm an A+ parent and some days I just get a passing grade. I felt that since I gave up my career to be a stay-at-home mom, I had to be the archetypal mother! Gradually, over the years I let go of the myth of doing it all. Parenting books didn't work for me. Their theories were good on paper, but they didn't work at home. My girls would say, 'Are you trying out something you read in a book?' Then on top of the stress of being a good parent, I felt pressured, as the oldest sibling, to be more attentive to my aging parents. In addition, I wanted my house to look neat and inviting and to be Martha Stewart in the kitchen. I finally realized that I just can't make everyone happy all the time. I had to take a step back and look at why I needed to please everyone around me."

The harder Joanne tried to please everyone, the more depleted and irritable she felt, the complete opposite of her goal to be the perfect nurturer. Ironically, Joanne's involvement with her daughters' religious education classes turned out to be the best remedy for her need to accommodate everyone. She learned by teaching her students that *God always loves us for what we are.* In other words, we are good enough already! There's a plan for why we are meant to be doing what we are doing, although we can't see the whole picture. It's a big adventure. When Joanne eased up on herself, she was able to flow with the current.

Contrast is the point of this story. Conceptualize it like this: you can *be calmly active and actively calm.* How can we appreciate what we have if we don't lose it at some point? In Catholicism the saints experience the agony and the ecstasy. In Judaism, the heavens are composed of powerful opposites, fire and water. In both religions, mankind is created in God's image, yet we are both mortal and immortal. Our pain and suffering lead to spiritual growth and development—and of course, further joy.

If stress is part of life and no one is to be spared, we owe it to ourselves to transform this nervous energy into strength. Let's take all this diffuse, anxious energy and use it to fuel a power plant! A little stress helps activate the immune system clearing away bacterial and viral invaders. Also, stress stimulates the mind to help us perform better on tests, on the job and in public performances. What we need to learn is how to channel the energy of stress into productivity and creativity, and then decompress.

Sr. Kathleen, a Coordinator of Human Services, explains that, "When things get really difficult, I draw inspiration from my favorite quote from Ralph Waldo Emerson: *Every person I meet is my senior.* To me the words mean that everyone has something to teach us, especially people who are difficult. At least, we can try not to be difficult ourselves." An added benefit is that in dealing with such people, she has to cultivate more internal patience. When she is calm, she can find another way, another approach.

Good Stress

Stress can help us to take action to find a solution when we receive bad news or a bad diagnosis. If we accept the disappointment with total equanimity, we might find ourselves feeling fatigued and sluggish, floating around distractedly. An objective observer might say that we are mildly depressed. The inability to act signals that we are feeling helpless. Eventually, we might become more helpless and accepting of whatever is being done to us, i.e., the sacrificial lamb. However, if we take our stress and use its energy to get a second opinion, another physician, or a support group, then we are channeling nervous energy into positive power. At this point our senses are on high alert; we have a balanced awareness of what is on the ground and likely to trip us up, and what is above, spiritually helping to lift us with an invisible string attached to the crown of our head.

A frantic daughter wrote to me that her mother, who was in the middle stages of Alzheimer's, accused her of stealing her medicine, insinuating that she was plotting to kill her. In fact, the daughter was so loving that she had moved from Alabama to Ohio to help her father cope with her mother's condition. Although she realized her mother was speaking from a diseased brain, the words stung. She did not know how to calm her mother's agitation and as a result grew more frustrated. Obviously she could not let her mother take charge of her own medication, as she would surely over- or under-medicate. I advised her to keep placebo pills in a different medicine bottle allowing her mother some semblance of control. She could be at ease knowing that her mother was safe from overdosing. I also advised her to be more creative with her mother. "Touch and hug her. Play the favorite tunes from her era. Don't be afraid to love her. Distract her with photographs or objects she enjoys when she gets upset. Don't argue your truth. See the truth with Alzheimer's eyes." There is always another way—a better way.

Another technique for turning stress into strength is to keep a journal. Sr. Diane Capuano uses this method for releasing stress by recording her story *as is:* "I journal a lot about my feelings, worries, experiences and whatever comes up. After I complete a journal, which usually contains about six months to a year's worth of experiences, I'll read through it to find the pattern; then I bless it and get rid of it. I note my growth experiences and times of trial, and then I move on and write the next chapter." For Sr. Diane objectifying the chapters of her life, reviewing them like an outside observer, a critic so to speak, and then discarding them, provides closure and enables her to move forward. Those of us who shudder at the thought of writing can speak into a tape recorder regularly, and then listen to it weeks or months later, analyzing what is being said as well as what is *not* being said.

Another alternative for transforming stress into strength is to intentionally reinterpret the conflict, the performance, or the diagnosis. Perception is within everyone's control. How do I choose to perceive the stressful situation that is draining me of life and energy? The most direct route towards emotional strength is retelling the story from another point of view. Take Hansel and Gretel, for instance. One version of the story stars two juvenile delinquents who torment their stepmother and run away from home to make her look bad. They encounter a senior citizen in the forest, and with great prejudice toward the elderly insult her by calling her a witch. Next, the two youths literally eat the woman out of house and home. Then Gretel, an innocent looking, fair-haired child, unexpectedly shoves the poor old woman into the oven! This perspective completely changes the dynamics of the charming story that's been passed down to us.

Perhaps we can reinterpret an insult or other offending event with love, compassion and forgiveness, letting go of our notion of being right, letting our need to be right fly up to the heavens where it absolutely belongs—to God. The fact is that none of us knows the absolute truth about others, or about ourselves, even when we think we do. We are complex beings with complex stories. Basically everyone has an ego and everyone wants to be right. Psychologist Carl Jung said: *"The shoe that fits us so well pinches the foot of another."* Perhaps we can give up the need to be right and to assert our truth, and live according to this theory of relativity.

You might think that nuns practice reinterpreting injustices automatically. Well, they are only human. They get angry and stressed by long days, needy people, obstinate co-workers and superiors, obeying orders they would like to see changed, living with other women and having their personal creativity restricted by the rules and the structure of convent life. Sister Kathleen shared a menacing moment that taught her the importance of letting everyone be right on some level.

"I have learned a lot about kindness and respect from one of our young male volunteers," she says. "One day a deranged homeless man came to us for help. However, there was a slight problem: he had a three-foot rusty machete! I was scared and upset. However, our male volunteer spoke to him respectfully and kindly, calming him down and most importantly listening to him. Basically, he accepted the homeless man in the place that he was in emotionally. The man handed him the machete as though he were handing over an umbrella. Our volunteer placed the machete under my desk at my feet, as if it were an offering. At that moment I realized how important it was to accept people on their own terms and to really listen to their personal truths."

If we are looking for guidance in reinterpreting negatives into positives, we can all learn from the Buddhist monks who incorporate this practice in their daily spiritual training. In fact, their daily mental exercises consist of conjuring up aggravating scenarios and reinterpreting them with positive perceptions. They are constantly rewriting stories.

Buddhists do this so often in their training that reinterpretation becomes reflexive. Stress is turned into strength of character and strength of purpose. No longer drained by negative energy, Buddhists are free to live in the present. By reinterpreting the past, you are free to create the present. When Buddhists' brains were analyzed by PET scans in a study conducted by the Harvard Medical School, the left prefrontal cortex, the part of the brain responsible for happiness and optimism, was active for the entire twenty-four hours. This means that Buddhists are happy and alive with positive energy when they are awake and asleep. In other words, Buddhists do it better!

Before you are able to reinterpret negatives into positives, however, it helps to first physically de-stress. Using your body's own resistance in a modest burst of physical activity is the most direct route for transforming stress into strength. The intensity is based on your own perception of your exertion level, because what is intense to you may be moderate to someone else. If you are busy throughout the day and do not have a block of time to dedicate to traveling to and from a gym, along with showering and changing, try another option, the Changing Habits program depicted in chapter 13. Two ten-minute intervals of resistance training a couple of times a day at home or work performing the demonstrated exercises and their variations, with or without weights, will literally inoculate you against the harsh realities of life.

The effectiveness of resistance training depends on perception. In an extreme example, bedridden stroke victims, who did not want their muscles to atrophy, visualized expanding and contracting their leg and arm muscles throughout the day. The result was startling. There was far less muscular atrophy for those who visualized than for stroke victims who did not image their muscles working. I can only conclude from this study that if we concentrate on the muscle that we are working, even without weights, there will be significant growth in muscle fiber, improved strength for functional fitness, and reduced stress. Focused attention on the working muscle will greatly enhance the physical results. An extra benefit is that focused attention redirects us from our worries to break the cycle of nagging thoughts.

One of my favorite turning-stress-into-strength exercises is playing catch with a medicine ball, which looks like a basketball and comes in weights ranging from two to fourteen pounds. Select a medicine ball, readily available in most sporting-goods stores, weight to be determined by you. If you're a beginner, for example, you'll probably want to start with a two- or three-pound ball. Find a partner and play a game of catch. However, this is not an ordinary game of catch because it involves reinterpretation.

When you throw the weighted medicine ball, think or say out loud: *"I throw off my negativity, my nervous feelings and my worries."* When it is your turn to catch, think: *"I catch the abundance that life has to offer."* After a few minutes, you will be laughing and feeling warm inside and out. Think it and do it. You're training yourself to feel better physically and mentally.

Throwing a weighted ball is aerobic. You build upper-body strength in the chest, shoulders, biceps and triceps. Women tend to have weaker upper bodies, and therefore this exercise is replete with health benefits, combining strength training with cardio fitness. If you don't have a partner for this exercise, then throw the ball up in the air and catch it. Throw it haphazardly, so that sometimes it comes down to the right and the next time to the left or farther afield. That will make you think of Divine energy and God's role in your life. Believing that you are good enough and that God is with you and within you will free you to take the first step to transforming stress into strength.

When you feel unsettled, anxious, angry or despondent, realize that you hold the ball in your hands. A hand is an emblem of both empowerment and benevolence. Its five fingers symbolize five basic instincts for happiness. You can count them on your fingers like a high five. The first is the *survival* instinct, the life force. The second is *choice*, the right to say no. The third is *empowerment*, the ability to make a unique contribution. The fourth is *social*, the power of friendship. The fifth is *fun*, releasing your inner child and cuting loose. Exercise strengthens you to grow healthier, more honestly expressive, more powerful, more charismatic and relaxed with your personal whims. Happiness is as simple, fun, and within your grasp as a game of catch. The more you practice, the better you get.

Self-care Mantras

- ◆ Ease up on yourself and flow with the current.
- ◆ Be calmly active and actively calm.
- ◆ The shoe that fits us so well pinches the foot of another.
- ◆ By reinterpreting the past you are free to create the present.
- ◆ Accept people on their own terms and listen to their personal truths.

Chapter 3

LIFT WEIGHTS TO LIFT YOUR SPIRITS

Many of us experience our daily routines with confused thinking, low frustration tolerance, the inability to make decisions and excessive worrying. The recent popular television show, *Desperate Housewives* (their husbands aren't too happy either), evokes Henry David Thoreau's quote: "Most people live lives of quiet desperation." As the show portrays, we look for an easy fix in the form of purchase power, pills, plastic surgery, and/or an affair. We want to believe the modern-day fairytale that more money will make us happy; plastic surgery will transform us into swans; a new romance will give us those butterflies that make us feel alive and excited with new possibility. However, even when our dreams come true, the initial distracting thrill wears off and the pendulum inevitably swings back to our original unhappy center. Why?

Basically, we have unrealistic expectations about our appearance, our love life and our finances. Even those who have had liposuction, botox, restylene and facelifts realize that the forces of gravity and time are far more powerful than a surgeon's medical tools. Once the surgery barrier is broken through, many women become addicted to fixing the never-ending crop of imperfections with more surgical intervention. Inevitably, the fat returns to the same places or is re-deposited in other areas. Thinking that we can revitalize our spirit and activate our joy simply by re-contouring and resurfacing the outside proves futile.

All of this dissatisfaction is based on our need to have it all. The great news is *that we can have it all—just not all at the same time!* If we make up our minds to be reasonably happy and to generate positive energy, we will freely attain that which we desire. Especially when we don't feel like it, we must *act as if;* then we will eventually become all that we aspire to become. We need to assume responsibility for what happens to us and *act* to release our true inner selves. The true self refers to the way we live in daily reality, not what we imagine we are or wish to become. For example, are there obligations in your life that you resent? Do you want to let them go? Liberate yourself this very moment! Think about one small thing you wish to change in your life like drinking more water or going to sleep thirty minutes earlier and do it now. If you are not sure about other things you wish to change in your life, keep a list of your daily needs and observe which ones you fulfill and which ones you don't. Make it a priority to address at least one personal need a day.

Do not be afraid to lift weights

Most of us would never consider weight lifting although it is a very effective path to both health and happiness. Many women balk at the notion of weight training and the biggest fear, bulking up and looking like a huge steroidal male body builder. Because of our hormone levels—mostly estrogen and relatively little testosterone—this is just not going to happen. However, weight lifting will help us do many wonderful things for both mind and body.

Weight lifting is a spiritual experience. You align your body, support your core, breathe through and ultimately execute the movement by focusing on the mind/muscle connection. You imagine what the muscle is accomplishing by isolating that part of your body and consciously sending your breath to that location. Each movement is slow and controlled and requires your full attention, to live in the now.

Weight training helps you live in the now

It is a blessing to be immersed in the present not worrying about the past or future. When lifting weights, your concentration is directed to your body executing what your mind is signaling it to do. In turn your body fully senses what it is doing and returns that signal to your mind. When you weight lift in this fashion without swinging the weights—because you are rushing to get it over with—you are engaged in a spiritual moment of total concentration.

All worries melt away. Problems do not exist at this time. Your attention is devoted to what your muscle is accomplishing. Your breathing works to oxygenate both your muscle and your brain. When you exhale upon exertion, you lower your blood pressure and rid the body of toxins.

The result over a period of time is concretely measurable using an easy-to-read blood pressure home kit. You can visibly see muscle growth and feel the strength you have accrued when lifting grocery bags out of the car or reaching up and putting away a heavy box on the top shelf. You can check your posture in the mirror and see how much taller and straighter you stand. Avoiding the tendency to be smug and coast, the next step is to use slightly heavier weights. The principle for weight lifting, as in life, is overload and adaptation. You stimulate the muscle to grow by taxing it a bit, and after adaptation you continue the process by moving on to the next level.

You can't change where you came from. However, you can change where you are going. Strength training can change where you are going and enhance the stability and determination in your steps to get there. Strength training exercises have contributed to my strong positive core and internal motivation. Because opposing muscle groups contract and relax at the same time to lift a weight, my body has taught me to tighten my spirit in order to never give up on myself, and at the same time to ease up and believe with *certainty* that life will work itself out as it is meant to.

However, sometimes we find it difficult to get motivated to work out, especially to lift weights. On those days we simply have to be determined to do it, to pull the intent out of ourselves, because we make strength training a part of our health routine and an integral part of our life.

Esther, a petite five-foot Kennedy Airport security guard, confides, "Sometimes I just don't feel like working out for whatever reason. But I know it's good for me and it is part of my routine. So, I drag myself to the gym and I begin. I tell myself that I don't have to go through my whole workout—I can do half. Half is better than nothing. Then after I do half, I tell myself I can do a little more. Before I know it, I do the whole thing and I feel better about myself."

Did you know there is a Kabbalistic story about the spirituality of strength training?

Once upon a time there was a great ladder suspended from heaven reaching all the way down to earth, but not quite touching. The lowest rung appeared to be almost within reach, yet no one had ever reached it. Everyone who perceived the ladder kept jumping higher and higher, trying to grasp the lowest rung. Time passed and finally one person jumped high enough and reached the rung. I am adding to the story this question: wouldn't it be wonderful if we could share our successes with one another and be interdependent? Together we would lift one of the jumpers to the lowest rung. Looking back down from the ladder of personal success, this person could then help form a human chain which would hoist one jumper at a time. Strength training will help us to develop the mentality to accomplish this physically and spiritually.

Studies show that people who begin strength training later in life discover that they are more willing to try exciting new activities. They are strong enough to step out of the box and explore new opportunities. Some are strong enough to break the box!

Why bother weightlifting when there are so many aerobics classes given?

The benefits of weightlifting are numerous:

◆ Stronger skeletal frame to reverse osteopenia (bone density loss) and prevent osteoporosis

◆ Greater muscle mass to protect the joints and prevent injury

◆ More efficient calorie burning for weight management

◆ Stronger back muscles for better posture

◆ Greater balance to prevent falls

◆ Better/Increased self-esteem

◆ More personal empowerment

◆ Improved concentration for mental tasks

It is important to note that what happens during a workout parallels what happens in the activities of daily living. Weightlifting helps you to get in touch with your body, to feel and control your bones, muscles and joints. When you control your body by responding comfortably to its signals, you exercise greater control over your life at home, at work and in your relationships.

Feel your body

To get in touch with your body try this simple change in perception when you lift weights: Hold a 2-3 lb. dumbbell in each hand and then bring both arms to shoulder height and lower to your sides. Lift and lower as you hold your weights. Now close your eyes and repeat this movement. Feel your bare bones lifting. Slowly perform this exercise with your eyes closed for a full set of 8-12 repetitions exhaling upon exertion. *Don't swing your arms.* Next, try this same move with your eyes open focusing on your muscle. Sense the change in your perception? You now have a better understanding of what weightlifting is all about. Also, your energy is not dissipated because you are in full contact with yourself! What I enjoy most about strength training is its demand for complete focus.

No distractions

However, I must confess that initially while I was lifting weights, I kept thinking about my appointments and the to-do list for the day. I kept looking anxiously at the clock. Suddenly, I glanced in the mirror and saw that my body was out of alignment; my grip was wrong and apparently, I was doing my body more harm than good at this point. Moreover, I wasn't holding my abdominals in tightly to support my back and I wasn't breathing properly through each move. If my trainer Frank Mikulka (you'll meet him and his fitness strategies in Chapter 13) was present, I would have never heard the end of it! Apparently, I wasn't the only transgressor at the gym. I did a quick check around the room and noticed a woman doing side leg lifts while speaking on her cell phone. She was just swinging her legs with her back rounded—all wrong!

Suddenly, I realized in a breakthrough moment that I must also be performing tasks at work distractedly. I was allowing my mind to wander to my mother's course of treatment in the hospital, my daughter's PSAT classes, my shopping list for the supermarket. I was accustomed and adept at multi-tasking, doing things rapidly—or so I thought. As a stress-management specialist, of course, I could handle it. However now I realized that I wasn't really giving it my all! Instead of saving time, everything took a little bit longer to do and everything was a little less than my best. The parallel was clear: I had sloppily and mechanically lifted weights during my workout and this cluttered mindset crept into my work without me realizing it. I had to stop bringing my mother, my daughter and *what are we going to do about dinner* to work with me. I had to simply do my workout and my work without distraction—what a relief!

When we strength train, it is helpful to channel our frustrations and stressors outward into the exercise not inward to ourselves. Before we begin a workout, we can have a logical discourse with ourselves, "I have some problems right now that I do not know how to solve, but at least I can exert control in my strength training." However, what if we do our best and it turns out that we are not successful in executing a particular exercise because we feel sad or overburdened? We don't need to let it dominate our whole performance. We don't need to say, "See, I'm a failure; I can't even do this right. Nothing is going right in my life!"

We can all learn from a pianist who plays a discordant note during her recital and gets past it by not allowing the error to dominate her whole performance which turns out to be brilliant. And isn't it the brilliant sounds that are always remembered, the whole effect, not the one or two discordant notes? On the contrary that error makes the pianist more human and triumphant because she is able to move past her mistake. Similarly, when we strength train, if our session wasn't perfect, we can get past it. When I'm not performing at my best or my energy levels are low, Frank reminds me, "We don't end on a note of failure. We end with our last success. See yourself going through the movement. Lift weights first mentally, then physically. Imagine that you are a champion, completing what you set out to do." Guess what? I can do it.

Become your own positive coach, not a negative one. What we say to ourselves influences what we believe we can do. Our words can create miracles or bring devastating effects. During our workouts we can practice getting into the habit of positive self-talk. When I speak positively to myself during my workout, I will speak positively to myself on the job, at home or with friends.

When we strength train, we can learn confidence-building tricks which correspond to life in general. Whenever we lose motivation and feel stuck, a change in our routine will work wonders. Sometimes adding a little weight, trying out a new fitness move or changing the order and the intensity help build confidence because we are trying something new without the pressure of a previous failure. When we succeed, past failures are erased from our minds and we feel renewed self-esteem and positive energy.

My weight training transgression led to a new resolution: I would not allow myself to be distracted from the activity of the moment. I would not divide myself, or more accurately, fragment myself, from what I was doing. Each time I weight trained, I reminded myself to be in the moment. Sometimes I had to close my eyes while I was doing abdominals or shoulder presses to really go inside myself and shut out distractions. I then trained myself to transfer this concentrated focus to all my duties, in order for my best and most creative self to emerge and not be diluted. Strength training taught me to operate at full strength!

As a result, weight lifting helped me to become more joyous. I permitted myself the personal time from a half hour to an hour each day to focus my mind fully on my muscles. Wonderful things happened over the course of a month. I made greater progress in physical strength and people in the gym asked me if I had liposuction! I accepted the remark as a strange compliment. In addition, I enjoyed this special time carved out purely for me. No worrying allowed! I created time to work on attainable goals without any accompanying anxiety, deadlines or guilt.

I transferred these newly acquired skills not only to my work and my home, but also to my friendships and relationships. When I had a conversation with someone, I listened with full attention, not thinking about what I would say while the other person was still talking. Since I was stronger, I felt more empowered. I didn't have to talk all the time because I was afraid of being invisible or ignored. As a result, people around me felt accepted and responded respectfully and kindly even when opinions differed. And I learned a great deal because I was truly present, listening to what was said and what was not said.

Connect to whatever you are doing

Sister Virginia, as the Prioress of the Sisters of St. Dominic Queen of the Rosary, does a great deal of listening. In fact, she carves out personal time for contemplation and exercise to make her a more effective listener, open to hearing everyone's truth and perspective. Exercising and meditating also enable her to speak her own truth. Because she has an extremely full calendar, she takes time to reset herself—to make sure that she is connected to whatever she is doing. Sister Virginia explains that healthy living connotes balance. When things get hectic, to restore her emotional balance, she asks herself: "Where am I? Where am I going? These questions help bring me back."

Exercise is not an all-or-nothing proposition

Also on the physical plane, Sister Virginia takes an almost daily mindful walk around the beautiful grounds of the convent with weights in her hands to recharge her mind and body. No one ever dictated that we have to use dumbbells only in a gym setting. Holding weights as she walks outdoors enables her to absorb the positive energy of nature—a synergy of mind/body/spirit. If Sister Virginia has meetings scheduled in different locations, she will park her car a few blocks from her destination and walk to squeeze in some exercise. She makes a point of taking the stairs instead of an elevator. These simple options do not make working out an all or nothing proposition. A little here and there add up. So if we experience stress at home or at work, ten minutes of weight training can rid us of stress hormones as it releases endorphins. The benefits are clear thinking and good health.

Sister Diane alternates her daily exercise regimen: one day it's a brisk two-mile walk with strength training for upper body and the next day it's pedaling on a stationary bike along with an abdominal workout. "I have learned to take this daily time to rejuvenate my body and to raise my spirit. If I have something stressful to do, not only do I pray and meditate, but I strength train. I have come to know my weaknesses and sense when my body is fatigued. I honor my body because I move with God's spirit. My responsibility is to stay healthy, to be attuned to God working through me. In my late twenties I lived with a great deal of pain, particularly lower back problems. Strength training my abdominals and doing back exercises with a chiropractor have helped me to achieve clarity and resonate with my duties. I don't get overwhelmed at work. I am strong enough physically and emotionally to pull myself out of it." Sister Diane explains her ability to stay centered, "I learned to focus on whatever I am doing."

In strength training a *loose* mind wastes energy. By tightening our minds we can focus our mental and physical energies, accomplishing more and not feeling as tired. As a result, we feel happier, positively energized and have more patience with those in our care. We can lift weights for many years, but if we merely go through the motions without directing our minds to the muscle, we will never experience the heart of the matter. Similarly, by not worrying or feeling anxious about completing the job at hand, but rather doing whatever we do with total immersion, we will feel at ease rejoicing in the completion of the task. Consequently, we grow more confident about the next challenge. Each success builds greater self-esteem equipping us with personal empowerment.

Ironically, resistance training will dissolve our resistance to lift weights. As our energy levels increase and our endorphins surge, we will experience a flash of clarity that will open us up to receive inspiration. Let us enjoy the glorious energy we generate from self-care and self-awareness—strengthening our muscles, bones, joints, heart and soul.

The human body is the only engine with the ability to improve its parts rather than wear out after continuous use. The principle is to do *just enough* demanding exercise and rest the next day. Gradually make the exercise a little more demanding to experience continuous and measurable improvement. That means: walk a little further, lift a little more weight or try a new exercise. Every time we explore a new physical skill, a whole new set of neuromuscular reactions are set into motion to create subtle changes in our mental alertness and in our confidence. Learning new physical skills keeps our brain growing and stimulated.

When we realize what we can accomplish with our physical strength because our minds are also moving that muscle and lifting that weight, we move beyond our personal doubts and fears. Although we don't bulk up the way men do, we do become larger than ourselves, more hopeful and capable of implementing our inspirations. We feel alive!

Self-care Mantras

- ♦ We can have it all—just not all at the same time.
- ♦ You can't change where you came from. You can change where you are going.
- ♦ We don't end on a note of failure; we end with our last success.
- ♦ Strength training teaches you to operate at full strength.
- ♦ Listen to what is said and what is not said.

Chapter 4

HAVE STRENGTH IN YOUR FAITH
AND FAITH IN YOUR STRENGTH

External strength partners internal strength in the same way that we partner our bodily health when we take vitamins or medications. Faith in God, Divine energy, partners belief in ourselves. *Time Magazine* (October 24, 2004) has validated our leap of faith with the discovery of the God gene: we are all programmed genetically to seek God. Scientists claim that we have a *spiritual* gene to help reduce the sting of our mortality through belief in the upbeat story of a higher power and a happy-ever-afterlife. Their take is that God is a neuro-chemical byproduct of the brain. Theologians smile knowingly and respond that this explanation is limited because spiritual genes are actually part of the Divine scheme of things—our individual journey to unite with God. This means that we can have faith in our strength and strength in our faith. In other words, our spirit and muscles are designed to work together: Conceive, Believe, Achieve. In the words of Muhammad Ali, a man possessing great physical strength, *Impossible is nothing!*

The mind is the powerful control center in everything we do. When we do not believe in ourselves, we tend to put up imaginary prison bars to keep us where we are. Negative thoughts and self-doubts can undermine whatever risks or changes we set out to try. The problem is that we keep hearing the old disparaging voices of childhood: "You just can't do anything right, can you?" "Why can't you be more like your sister?" "You're so irresponsible." "I'm not going to buy you a new dress until you lose some weight." Because of these past judgments, we sentence ourselves to a life filled with mediocrity and settle into prescribed roles of accommodating others—saying yes when we really mean no—in order to be liked and complimented. We keep busy to choke down our dreams and our needs. We feel guilty if we make time for ourselves because fundamentally we believe that we are not worth it. After all we are accustomed to suppressing our desires and creative expression.

Common symptoms of a lack of self-confidence

- ◆ You feel anxious about mingling at a party wondering if anyone will talk to you or if you will say anything engaging.
- ◆ You repeatedly check your appearance in the mirror and reapply makeup or tug at your clothes as you pull in your stomach.
- ◆ You fail at something you worked on and can't shake that feeling of inadequacy. Your failure has assumed your identity.
- ◆ You feel that you have been victimized and take no responsibility for being fired or divorced.
- ◆ You feel guilty about changing your doctor even when the doctor proves to be incompetent or continually ignores you when you try to explain your symptoms.

All these symptoms point to a common denominator: you are lacking self-confidence. Unfortunately knowing that you lack self-confidence does not make you feel any better about yourself!

Most daily stressors gnaw at the root of self-esteem; filling your mind with perceived enemies and old conflicts drains your spirit and saps your creative joy. However, no one can trivialize you, label you, or crush your convictions if you know and accept who you are.

Don't let so-called friends talk you down

When I reinvented myself into a new career path leading to stress-management workshops, writing and radio show hosting, some people tried to chip away at my creativity and confidence; in fact, a close girlfriend tried to destabilize my motivation: "Who are you to do this? Stick to what you know and do best—gardening." A couple of months later I was told by a social worker from a prestigious medical center that I wasn't important enough to address her group. I found this remark particularly ironic since social workers generally uplift and encourage others. Did I waver? Well, perhaps just a little bit, but because I am passionate about what I do and believe that the harder I work, the better I get, I dug my heels into the earth. Gradually, I distanced myself from toxic friends who tried to undermine my resolve with a simple, unemotional statement: "I don't have time to talk now, got to go." Basically, I learned from my mistakes, studied more, listened more and believed more than ever and with greater certainty in myself.

Only six short months later I addressed an auditorium filled with several hundred people. One woman called out to me as I was making my way to the podium. I will never forget her words: "You look like someone important. Are you today's speaker?" I smiled and responded, "We are all important." She nodded and said, "I think I'm going to enjoy today's program." To this day I believe her words were a sign giving me a heads up.

Take back your power

As much as I would love to, I can't give you the power to see yourself in a positive, capable light. You have to assume that power on your own; stand up for yourself and know what you uniquely bring to the table of life. Next, you have to value your contribution and see it as distinct from everyone else's. If you don't know what your gifts are, try the following empowerment exercise.

Empowerment Exercise

This quick exercise will bring you closer to positive self-awareness. Think back to a time when you were successful—something concrete that you achieved. Consider an accomplishment that was clearly validated by others and quantifiable as a success. I do not mean an achievement which you have to interpret metaphorically as a victory; rather, an accomplishment that has been objectively praised. Once you have recalled this triumph, write a *shopping* list of all the personal qualities you pulled together to make it happen. Review your list to see in black and white what special traits in your personality shine through. Once you have identified those qualities, transfer them to your present activities of daily living. How can you incorporate these good traits into making you happier and healthier today?

In one of my stress-management workshops, we set aside fifteen minutes to do this exercise. Michelle's example stands out as representative of the group. Michelle remembered returning to school after ten years of married life to graduate with an Associate's Degree and a 4.0 index. She itemized the following traits which contributed to her success: *time management, concentration* and *entitlement.* At the time Michelle was busy raising two young children. She carved out time for herself two nights a week which became known as *Pizza Nights.* The children understood and accepted that she would be immersed in her school work. Michelle then applied focused *concentration* to study the material—a martial artist would have envied her concentration! With each "A" her confidence rose. Finally, she felt *entitled* to those high marks and believed that she could achieve an "A" in every class. Most importantly, she believed that she deserved the personal time and space to improve herself and grow.

Currently, Michelle is being treated for thyroid cancer. She takes care of an ailing husband who is housebound and negative. They remain married because of her loyalty—"That's the way I was raised." In addition, two days a week she helps her daughter-in-law by taking care of two highly active pre-school grandchildren. No wonder Michelle's metabolism has suffered! Her cancer has lodged in the thyroid which controls metabolic function. She has been running on high energy, full throttle as a caregiver.

When Michelle first came to my workshops, she was worn out. She sat silently observing the others with her intense dark eyes. However, around the third session, she felt comfortable with the group and openly shared her problems and basic unhappiness. She confided that the 90 minutes she spent with our support group was the only time she took for herself and the only time she laughed out loud. "I turned off my cell phone and did not give my husband an emergency number because he would call for any silly excuse to rob me of my time here with my friends."

Imagine how powerful saying those three successful traits out loud—*time management, concentration and entitlement*—were for Michelle and the rest of us. My eyes met Michelle's. She realized at the very moment when she articulated those words, that she breathed an independent life into them. She gave them a distinct reality of their own. Michelle believed that she could use those same traits that helped her to earn high marks for an Associate Degree to take positive steps to reduce the stress and sadness in her life. She was determined to create daily personal time from 8:00 to 8:20 a.m. to meditate with scented candles and music. After all, she began to understand that she was entitled to it. The relaxation response lasted throughout the day slowing her down in her hectic lifestyle. Now when she gets too busy to meditate, her husband reminds her to do it!

The key to health and happiness is the balance between giving and receiving. If it is a blessing to give, then let other people share that blessing and give to us. When we are out of balance emotionally, we feel drained of positive energy and unsure of ourselves. As a result we feel irritable and push too hard to be better, but in the wrong direction. Instead of resting or doing something fun for ourselves, we try even harder to be accommodating and helpful because we need the addictive fix of other people complimenting us and boosting our self-esteem: "Wow, you're unbelievable!" or "You're a saint!" Unlike a saint, we do not feel connected spiritually because we are depleted and have lost our vitality for living. If we continue this lifestyle, we will likely suffer from physical ailments like chronic fatigue syndrome or auto-immune disorders. Auto-immune ailments are truly the *self against the self.*

You might be depressed and don't know it!

Mary Z confided that she experienced a bout of depression when her children were little, "It took six months for me to realize that I was depressed. I had to push myself to drive my daughter to choir practice on Sunday. I began to see a pattern. I was tired all the time. I was going through the motions like a robot. The only time I felt good was during Mass. Receiving Holy Communion was like taking a mood-elevating medication. So what was I going to do: leave the family, stop going to work and sit in church seven days a week, or go to a doctor? All this time I tried to stay cheerful and grateful for everything. I went around smiling and pretending everything was fine. After all, I had always been a cheerful person.

"My husband saw right through the façade. He felt that my cheerfulness wasn't real, that I was afraid to confront myself and that I was hiding and acting as if life was a wonderful, tap-dancing Broadway musical. It took some time, but I realized that he was right. I was suppressing my true feelings."

Mary was living a life of quiet desperation and she began to experience what was ultimately diagnosed as anxiety attacks. "I felt depleted. I realized that I was always running around.

Running away was closer to the truth because I really didn't want to sit and think. I was always cleaning the house, but the house was never clean—that sort of thing."

Mary decided to take a low dosage anti-depressant. She felt as though she had failed and was a weak person for taking a pill. However, the medication worked and she felt good again.

"So many people have anxiety attacks. It's not a stigma anymore. I opened up about it to my friends and realized that I wasn't the only one. Panic and anxiety are quite common. Currently, I'm off the pills. I'm not frightened anymore if my heart beats a little fast, if I feel pressure on my chest or have trouble breathing. I know what it is, what triggers it and I know what to do. I make time for myself. I love reading and I always learn something that helps me. I don't try to do everything. I ask for help. Also, I meditate, do deep breathing exercises and work out sporadically. Exercise is the first to go when I get busy. Every month I have a women's night out and experience a real sense of community; we discuss everything and my friends are really helpful!"

Mary's journey led her to develop faith in her own strength. She was strong enough and honest enough to confront her anxiety and her constant *busyness*. Most importantly, she realized that it was not a sign of weakness to feel anxious or panicky. Rather it was a sign of weakness to suppress and pretend that it didn't exist and that everything was fine. Mary has made it a top priority to exercise and has incorporated yoga postures to help her feel more centered and to stabilize her emotions.

Exercise stabilizes our emotional ups and downs

To activate our vitality for living we need to exercise. It is difficult or even impossible to maintain an exercise regimen if we hate to work out. We need to discover what kind of movements we enjoy and create a happy environment with upbeat music.

If you *still* hate exercising, examine the reasons why to expose the root cause of your sadness and anxiety:

♦ Ashamed of your body
♦ Afraid of being in you. ody because it houses some painful memories
♦ Fear of failure—if you don't try, you can't fail
♦ Comparing yourself to others

To help you have faith in your own ability you need to look at things differently: perceive exercise as self-healing, grounding and generating positive energy. This means experimenting with different videos, checking out fitness magazines, trying new classes in a gym or community center to find the workout that makes your heart sing. A workout that wakes you up when you feel fatigued will keep you motivated to stay with it. Finally, change is important when you exercise. The body needs stimulation just like the mind, so try to introduce variety in your routine. Chart your muscular growth and quantify the improvements to see in black and white that you are getting better. Consider a workout to be a series of holy moments. We are strengthening the body to house the spirit.

Push off with the push-up

One of the best strength training exercises, easily doable anywhere, yet a bit intimidating for women is doing a push-up which uses the body's own resistance. This is a total upper body workout and is generally more difficult for women than for men who have greater upper body strength. There are three versions of this exercise: off the wall, off the knees and full body. All three postures work pectorals, triceps, biceps, shoulders and abdominals. This is an exercise that you build up slowly. You can actually feel and see the muscular development. Nevertheless most women dread the push-up.

Push-ups have been a difficult strength-training move for me as well. My trainer Frank Mikulka, demonstrating a Changing

Habits push-up in chapter 13, pointed out that my upper body was definitely strong enough to do a full body push-up as evidenced by the weight I bench-pressed. Yet I was afraid that my arms would not support my body. I resisted this observation, but later that day I did think about the fear angle. You know the old story how for a few weeks one whispers into the king's ear, in this case the queen's, and suddenly the royal one remarks, "I just had an idea!" Well that was me. Frank was right and only a man who understood fear on a profound level, who had confronted and faced fear, would sense it on the training floor. That's the stuff a good trainer or a good life coach is made of.

This helps prove an important premise: What happens during a workout and what we learn about ourselves during that workout translates into activities of daily living. There is a vital connection between what we believe and how our body responds. In a later workout when Frank instructed me to do some push-ups, inside my head I kept repeating, "My arms can support me. I can do this push-up in good alignment and go all the way down and back up again. My arms won't break." Then I prayed that it would be over soon. "Excellent, Debbie! Do you know that you did 17 push-ups perfectly! That's enough to pass part of the physical fitness test in the Police Academy. One cadet I worked with passed everything else with flying colors, except that she couldn't do those 17 pushups, but you can!"

What made all the difference in a week's time? I didn't suddenly become Samson. However, I had faith in my strength, in my personal empowerment. I knew that if I didn't quit on the training floor, then I wouldn't quit in real life.

I still don't like doing push-ups, but I hate them less than I did. I know that I can do them and I know that they are good for me. They help me to open my heart and not be afraid of being vulnerable or rejected. They help me to believe in myself that I can go the distance when I face my fear and persist. Small steps, giant gains.

Sr. Peggy shares how she generates self-confidence: It is about being true to yourself and to your potential. "Self-confidence requires a quantum leap of faith in yourself. Meditation helps reacquaint ourselves with our spirit." If you are too busy and restless to sit still and meditate, Sr. Peggy suggests taking what she calls a *Thanksgiving walk.* After a recent Thanksgiving Day dinner, feeling sluggish, she took a brisk walk in her neighborhood and became inspired. She decided that the theme of her holiday fitness walk would be good for all seasons—out into the light in praise of the self: body parts that have served us well all these years, our special character traits and accomplishments. For example: I am grateful that my heart, back, arms and legs are strong enough to shovel the snow to clear the path or I am grateful that I stopped to think and reinterpreted a conflict with a positive spin, letting go of my resentment. We will get many benefits from a *Thanksgiving walk:* generate good energy with exercise, absorb light energy and create time and space to be grateful for our good attributes. It becomes a multisensory experience proven to restore happiness.

Generate faith in yourself

The secret to getting **ahead** is getting **started:**

- ◆ Write down your goals to objectify and specify them. Often, we don't really think until we write.

- ◆ Express who you are by letting your inner self out! Dress the way you want and put on less make-up, or more if you don't wear any. Wear what is comfortable and makes you feel good.

- ◆ Close your eyes and visualize the successful completion of your goals. Believe that things will work out. See yourself successfully completing one goal after another. Rehearse the steps in your mind, so that you become proficient.

- Shoo away the bullies in your mind who eagerly provide the reasons why you *can't, shouldn't* and will ultimately fail. Nothing is impossible to a willing mind.

- Find friends who will serve as your life coaches to inspire you to victory. You need a nurturing environment to grow. Imagine a sports team whose coach told them they were no good. Ultimately the team would lose and the coach wouldn't have a job.

- If you fail, then assume responsibility. Learn from your mistakes and don't blame anyone else because then you give away your power. Victims are helpless. Don't let anger control you and defeat you.

- You don't have to excel at everything. Find the something you do well and build on it. Let that something be your identifying success.

- Become so strong inside that you do not have to demonstrate your power. It is a part of you, readily observable in your stance with shoulders back, heart open and head erect.

Be proud of yourself everyday. The giant oak is an acorn that held its ground.

Self-care Mantras

- Conceive, believe, achieve.
- Know what you bring to the table of life.
- The key to health and happiness is the balance between giving and receiving.
- The secret to getting ahead is getting started.
- There is a vital connection between what we believe and how our body responds.
- We can have faith in our strength and strength in our faith.

Chapter 5

MOVEMENT THAT MATTERS

When we hit a wall because the people and projects in our life aren't working out the way we planned, we tend to apply more force. Frustrated, we take it up a notch, pushing even harder for success. The reality is that forcing an issue does not get good results. Getting caught up in the frenzy of seeking to control, we thrash around as though caught in a riptide dangerously being pulled under. Ironically, all we have to do is to swim sideways a few feet away to safety and freedom and flow with the current.

Flowing means creating balance in body, mind and spirit. To stabilize ourselves, sometimes we have to let the current carry us—yielding to that which we cannot control and trusting in ourselves and others. We can break up our life into moments and be satisfied with the moment. If a particular moment is frustrating, the next moment could be better. Sometimes we need to do absolutely nothing but wait and collect our energies. We might have to give up our preconceived plans, take a detour, or feel our way around intuitively.

When we flow, we become one with what we are doing, and we are graceful: Like a golf swing that emanates naturally from the golfer without his mind breaking up the swing into a series of prescribed movements. When we don't flow, it's like learning to dance. We concentrate so hard on getting it right, that our movements are forced; we forget to have fun.

Many of us are frustrated trying to control life partners, elderly parents and children—perhaps all at the same time. Although we mean well—"We know what's good for them," we have to respect the will and flow of others. Like love, we cannot compel, but instead, we set love free like a bird and hope that it flies back to us. Jacob M. Broude aptly summarized what we all need to take to heart when the urge to change others arises, "Consider how hard it is to change yourself, and what little chance you have of trying to change others."

Ease up and learn how to flow

- ◆ If you are forcing an issue and are not successful, take a break for awhile. Trust that success will come to you from a power beyond yourself. Believe in a success that is much larger than yourself.

- ◆ Sit quietly in a natural setting and tap into your peaceful, loving self. Feel how large and infinite your spirit is. Absorb the landscape, whether an ocean, a garden, or a picture. Intuitive thoughts will flow freely and inspire you. They will come to you, sometimes in a dream.

- ◆ Play music that revitalizes and inspires you. Music provides the necessary stimulus to induce *flow*.

- ◆ Say *no* to activities or people who rob you of your quiet, relaxed time.

- ◆ Surround yourself with positive people to build up your energy level. We all absorb energy from others. Be careful and make sure to identify what kind of energy you absorb. Your movements in life will depend on it.

- ◆ Be patient with your goals. Tackle small, manageable goals. See what's right in front of you and immerse yourself in it and appreciate this small accomplishment. Ease up on a deadline for your grand vision. A deadline is exactly that—a *dead* line.

- ◆ As things unfold, flow with the changes and accept different directions, criticism and detours along the way. You might find greater success and happiness than you originally envisioned.

The origin of flow: Two heads are better than one

Basically, we have two brains: the cognitive and the limbic. For optimal performance they have to both get along! The cognitive brain houses the rational mind which is analytical and geared to society—what other people will think and say. The limbic brain is the primitive seat of emotions. It is instinctual and primarily concerned with survival, seeking to establish balance and searching for satisfaction. The limbic brain is involved with bodily functions particularly our response to stress, danger and gratification. While the cognitive brain can objectively analyze, interpret and rationalize life patterns and conflicts, the limbic brain is connected to feelings so deep that we cannot verbalize them.

To live in a state of flow we need to be in harmony with both our brains: rational and instinctual. No matter how much we want to rationalize our feelings away, they will return to haunt us through the body's signals. Oscar Wilde said in one of his offbeat witty epigrams. "Everything can be rationalized, even the truth!" However, our innermost feelings—the ones that cannot be put into words are more honest and enduring. Whenever we express our feelings, even the most intense, our rational minds can potentially distort them to fit our personal agenda. We can think up many good reasons to stay in an abusive relationship or in an unfulfilling career even though we feel fatigued, experience frequent headaches, a queasy stomach and feel vaguely unhappy.

To bring our two brains into a state of flow we need to connect the mind with the body. Specific exercises can serve as physical affirmations directly corresponding to life's challenges, personal doubts or spiritual needs. These exercises involve both brains. The principle is holistic: *Think it and do it.* For example: Pick up a medicine ball—available at most sporting goods stores—(weight to be determined by you from two to twelve pounds) and stand back to back with a partner. Pass the ball to each other in a continuous circular motion. You become one as you synchronize your movements to work in harmony. Continue to pass and receive the ball with one hand up on top and the other under the ball. Aim for twenty-five repetitions. Not only does this exercise work your obliques to give you a more tapered waist, but it also works your upper body and is aerobic. Subliminally, you are learning the art of compromise and team work responding to the pressure of your partner's touch. Also, you are learning to subtly assert yourself.

The movements become self-hypnotic potentially bringing about cognitive changes that are positive and joyous when we practice them. These movements easily transfer to daily life situations. Because we rehearse them on two levels with our rational mind and our physical body, they are transformed into natural, spontaneous and reflexive energy during stressful situations. When we get to the point where we can just perform the movements without having to think about them and are permeated with a sense of well-being, we flow as both brains are in sync. The result is that our minds and bodies feel relaxed and happy which is the key to good health.

Exercise heightens our senses to pleasure

When we perceive our specific exercise regimen as movement that matters, our positive emotional responses are reinforced which in turn motivate us to keep up the good work. We enjoy the good feelings and the energy boost. Exercise has a direct and powerful impact on the emotional brain. In fact, the more we exercise, the more receptive and heightened our senses become to all pleasures. People who exercise regularly actually delight in the little things in life: a savory bite to eat, a fragrance, a beautiful tree, a kind word or a hobby. By establishing regularity in an exercise program, we are less likely to experience anxiety attacks that overtake us by surprise. We find that problems have solutions.

In one of my workshops Francine revealed how making a conscious decision to exercise saved her sanity. At the time she was going through a painful divorce—if that wasn't bad enough—her daughter died of a drug overdose. Francine only saw the dark thunder clouds and who could blame her. It seemed to her that she had never lived her life. She moved into a small furnished apartment after she divorced, but was afraid to live there by herself since she considered the neighborhood a bit rough. Her physical condition made her feel even more vulnerable as she was a smoker and a couch potato. "I wouldn't have been able to run away from any attacker; I felt so winded from smoking!" Depleted and frustrated, she decided to change her life. She started walking regularly and threw away her last pack of cigarettes. As she built up her stamina, she began to alternate walking with jogging. "I enjoyed running—not running away, but running toward something."

Francine wanted to pick up the pace, but sometimes she couldn't run more than a couple of miles. She joined a runner's club for support and enjoyed it. She began to lift weights, run regularly with other members and to eat healthy nutrient dense foods. She loved the way her body felt—alive and well. She became increasingly aware of the trees and the scenery and how the sun felt on her skin. She ran a 13-mile race into a new life. Currently, she is remarried and happy. "At the time I knew that I was running for my life!"

When Sr. Peggy turned fifty-five, she turned a significant corner in her life. She decided that she would not trudge into mid-life by putting on a few extra pounds every year which would gradually sneak up and overwhelm her with a difficult-to-manage weight problem. Realizing that her metabolism was slowing down, even though her work wasn't, Sr. Peggy decided that she needed to change a few habits.

Walking by the beach was wonderful and meditative; however, her body had adapted to this regimen and it was not burning enough calories. She needed to incorporate strength training in her exercise program to surprise her body, speed up her metabolism as well as increase muscle mass. "I reasoned the whole purpose of exercise this way. When I counsel parishioners or deliver the homily, my body can't look out of balance or appear stooped with rounded shoulders. My demeanor and my posture represent my faith and carry an important subliminal message to parishioners. I put my mind and body into my work. If I ignore my body or don't take care of it properly, my message is weakened. It is my moral responsibility to maintain good health and physical strength to carry out my spiritual work. Lifting weights, walking briskly and water aerobics, all these different activities strengthen my body which houses my spirit. These movements matter to me. Even as I grow older, because of all my experience and education, I can still be ignited with creativity during what could possibly prove to be the best years of my life. I don't want my body to break down; I need it to support my mission and my spirit."

When I created the AAA (Activity Alleviates Anxiety) program for the sisters, I took note of which movements released feelings and associations; in other words, what resonated the most for them. For eight repetitions they did side laterals; they lifted their arms straight out to shoulder height and then lowered them to their sides. Although the movements were executed slowly and with control, I broke even this little bit of momentum by having the sisters hold this posture for ten seconds in the iron cross position. Then they did eight more repetitions and again held their arms out for ten seconds. Everyone experienced a burn without using any weights, but by using the body's own resistance which was more powerful than they had originally imagined. This exercise provided a good release of the daily responsibilities they shouldered.

Mind that muscle

When you mind your muscle, it grows and develops to a greater extent than if you were exercising while thinking about other things in your life. Many of the sisters felt invigorated by the *iron cross* position because they felt as though their shoulders were capable of releasing their burdens. They let all that tension ooze out of their bodies as they simultaneously strengthened their shoulders to carry out their missions. Then rolling their shoulders forward and back to relax and stretch the muscles that were just worked, the sisters sighed in relief. They felt at ease and strong.

The point of a *mind the muscle workout*, delineated in chapter 13, is to train you to carry out your duties without internalizing other people's tensions or absorbing their negative energy. Sister Maureen who is a social worker explains, "I have to set boundaries with the people I counsel because I will absorb their energy. I have learned to set those boundaries and to be playful. I make time to play by walking on the beach or calling up a friend and having a good laugh." That's wonderful advice as many of the mothers in my workshops have yet to set boundaries with their children.

Another movement which is a particular favorite in the convent and which never ceases to bring a smile to Sr. Grace's face is the dead-lift which culminates in the resurrection posture. The dead-lift is performed stiff-legged to strengthen the hamstrings and lower back, but with soft knees, because we never hyperextend a joint. In a standing position, legs shoulder width apart, abdominals tight, bend from the waist to achieve a flat back with eyes looking straight ahead for good body alignment. Focus your eyes straight ahead. Your back is like a table top and we could put a plate on it if we wanted to. Your arms hang down as though they were holding an imaginary bar. Slowly and gracefully rise from this bent position with your hands, palms facing down, sliding up the knees and thighs to stand straight and tall. Then raise your arms and extend them overhead, pulling your arms back slightly behind your ears. "And so I rise" we all say. Sister Grace glows when we do this posture with the accompanying words. The message is clear: we move from adversity to lightness of being. Although we are challenged by adversity, we advance in strength and spirit. From a *dead lift* to an *uplift* this strength training move gives shape and depth to recognizing an important principle of happiness: to free the self from the painful past.

We conclude the session with some balance exercises. One is a posture I adapted from yoga—I like to call it, the *Tree of Life*. Start by standing tall, shoulders back and both feet planted firmly on the ground. Balance on one leg as you turn your hip out with your foot flat against the supporting leg either at the ankle, the calf or the thigh. When the lower body is stable, move the arms together to form the prayer position which is an isometric hold: palm to palm. Gradually lift the arms up fully extended overhead palm to palm. Hold this position and breathe through it. Switch sides. I remind everyone to "find your personal balance between earth practicality and spiritual vision." Usually one side is visibly stronger than the other and that side can vary depending on daily activities. This posture presents alternatives based on personal ability. Most of the sisters maintain the position at the ankle level, a few of them at the calf and one or two at thigh level. This is a powerful centering and healing posture. The Tree of Life stands as the potent core of Jewish mysticism, the Kabbalah.

Do it; think it; choose wisely

During our weekly wellness workshop it was apparent to everyone in the group that Megan was doing much better. Her experimental treatments for melanoma were working. She felt quite strong and was still exuberant from a recent vacation where she swam with the dolphins, holding on to their natural force. She was determined to live her life fully.

During our session we discussed various mind/body strategies to boost the immune system as flu season was imminent. Then we did a few yoga stretches which included the Tree of Life posture to concretize the healing message. I concluded our time with a healing visualization and asked if anyone wanted to share any specific images that had surfaced. Megan wiped away tears. "My vision was beautiful. I saw a huge golden tree with long widespread branches. Standing beneath its branches, I felt safe and protected. Impulsively, I plucked one of its golden leaves and put it into my breast pocket. And then something magical happened. I was about to hug the tree to absorb its special energy. But instead, the tree hugged me with its golden branches. The tree was human in its embrace." The group interpreted the vision as a sign of healing for Megan. As we hugged her, we tapped into her glowing energy. Each of us was open to the power that flowed through her.

Our ability to flow in our relationships and in our bodies depends on the honest recognition of our conflicts and problems. What is the common denominator? Is it anger? The need to control? The need for recognition? The victim syndrome? Inner freedom comes to us easily when we both see and sense what is honest, that we are ready to assume complete responsibility for what happens to us. Our bodies help us to intuit the truth—but we must choose to listen and act.

Strength training the body by minding each muscle and appreciating what it does for us provides a major step in getting to know and feel the body. Tapping into our muscles enables us to infuse them with our spirit. When the movements are connected to an affirmation, our emotional well-being soars. A push-up is no longer a dreaded move executed to the thundering voice of a drill sergeant. Rather we perceive a push-up for what it really is: our upper body muscles working in unison to help us push off the ground and open our hearts to others. We are independent and responsible for coordinating our actions.

Perhaps, we can readily accept this interpretation of the push-up, but cannot imagine what is spiritual and flowing about a squat? Consider how many different lower body muscles we recruit when we execute a squat: ankles, calves, quadriceps, hamstrings, glutes, hips and abdominals—our total lower body. In this compound move we are strengthening our legs *to walk to their next happiness.* Squats enable us to spring out of a chair or ease on down the road. Our center, around our navel, is fortified. We are improving our balance and stance. And when we are centered, we know who we are and no one can knock us down. Our force is derived from the earth rooted in our legs rising up into our core. Everything emanates from that center; our arms and legs are as strong as our core like the branches of a tree are as strong as the trunk to which they are attached.

When we work out, we know that our muscles move purposefully. We realize that each movement has an impact on our emotional well being, yet we are probably unaware of how profound that impact is. If we are not concentrating, because we are executing the movement in a sloppy fashion or while speaking on a cell phone, then we might observe this *loose mind* carry over into our daily lives. However, when we are focused, mindful of each move and try our best to make each one count, we will see this level of concentration transfer to all our relationships and involvements! At the very least we will feel empowered and at ease, distracted from our worries and in touch with our core—our internal primal self. Then we are ready to flow in whatever we do. Like water, which always finds its path, we will gather our energy and either rise over obstacles or go around them and know as Rainier Maria Rilke said, "How deep is the reservoir from where our life flows."

Self-care Mantras

♦ If this moment is frustrating, the next moment could be better.

♦ To flow we need to live in harmony with both our brains: rational and instinctual.

♦ Exercise has a direct and powerful impact on the emotional brain.

♦ Our bodies help us to intuit the truth—but we must choose to listen and act.

♦ Strengthen your legs to walk to their next happiness

Chapter 6

WHAT IS THE CONDITION
OF YOUR HOUSE?

⚜

W e are bombarded with seductive ads, reality TV shows about marrying a prince-like millionaire, movies and pop songs persuading us that beauty and youth are all that matter. Beauty has become a skimpy one-size-fits-all mentality. Credit cards encourage us to shop for the latest styles, many of which are actually the old styles recalled to life with different buttons or a slight variation on the sleeves. Some of us are impulse-driven by the temporary high we get when shopping—only to return home feeling guilty. With a mad dash to reach the bedroom closet, we devise clever schemes that James Bond would have envied, to hide the price tags from our husbands who, if they ever find out, will chide us like silly school girls.

That's only the beginning. To measure up to what we buy, we starve ourselves to become the biggest losers in the lucrative weight-loss industry and often yo-yo between two states of being. We strut around wearing the emperor's new clothes pretending that we are quite comfortable tugging at our low-rise jeans that fit us like plumbers' pants hoping that we never have to sit down without our backs facing the wall. Simultaneously, we focus attention on our lines, wrinkles and cellulite. We buy expensive beauty products that promise a facelift in a bottle or drink supplements that are guaranteed to reverse the clock and smooth out our skin. When one beauty product falls short of its promises, we move on to buy the next one with a smiling young face on the box.

And here's the rub. The best-kept beauty secret is health and vitality. No matter how expensive and gorgeous our clothes are, no matter how much jewelry we wear or how our special make-up is applied, if we are not healthy or alive with positive energy, we will not look attractive. To look great we have to feel relaxed and at ease with our body—the look of contentment. How do we achieve this peace when life slams us with one stressful event after another? No need to purchase anything. As the saying goes, *the best things in life are free.* The answer is contained in our home.

Each one of us has been entrusted with a home. Some of us live in apartments or ranches; others in bi-level and even multi-level constructions; a few of us have some storage space in the attic. Some homes are brand new; while others are hand-me-downs from generation to generation. Our homes differ in appearance, condition, furniture, landscaping and location. Like any homeowner, we tend to match up to our neighbor's layouts, always evaluating market value, improvements and the all important location. At this point you might see the parallel to a metaphorical house, the body, and we don't have to belabor the obvious symbolism that it comes in all shapes, sizes, ages and conditions.

Are we happy with our homes? Are we content with the dwelling place of our spirit? I have never met a woman who has ever admitted, "I am beautiful, or I feel beautiful. I love myself just the way I am. There isn't a thing about me I would change." For that matter I meet few women who graciously accept a compliment with a simple, "Thank you." Instead, they qualify the compliment with excuses why they really don't deserve the compliment. On one level they are right. We did not choose our bodies—we were born that way—and we should not take full credit or criticism for the genetic results. However on another level, we can take credit for how we continue to support our frame, fix the plumbing, and of course, create our personal style.

Like any home that needs work, we can do a superficial job with mirrors, faux painting or wallpaper to hide the imperfections. We can choose to ignore the things that we don't see like termite damage, a leaky roof, old plumbing and wiring. However, eventually the structure will collapse as the skeletal frame disintegrates. No amount of *make-up* can restore or cover up a structural crack.

Your home has four rooms

Every home has four basic and necessary rooms; they are the rooms where we really live. All the rest of the space in our home can be considered fanciful extensions of these four rooms. In order to be healthy, energetic, confident and happy, we need to visit each of the four rooms of our home daily. The rooms are: the physical, the emotional, the intellectual and the spiritual. If we visit only one or two rooms, then we are not living in balance or in complete happiness. When we visit all four rooms, we can enjoy each room for what it has to offer—four distinctly different experiences every day.

The physical room

The physical room corresponds to the bodily processes. This room is simply furnished, actually skeletal. Here we become aware of what robs us of energy and what restores our energy.

Energy Drains:

♦ Sedentary lifestyle
♦ Diet replete with sugar, processed foods, caffeine, alcohol
♦ Skipping meals, particularly breakfast
♦ Dehydration
♦ Lack of sleep
♦ Environmental toxins
♦ Stress
♦ Toxic friends

Energy Boosters:

- Exercise
- A balanced diet of protein, complex carbohydrates and fat—preferably six small balanced meals a day
- A healthy breakfast
- Drinking about 8 cups of water a day
- Adequate sleep
- Controlling environmental toxins: Avoiding pesticides, opening the windows for fresh air, removing the plastic wrap over clothes that come from the cleaners and airing them out.
- Reinterpreting negatives into positives

Let's take a look at what keeps our bodily processes running smoothly. When we eat right, we send a nourishing message to both body and soul, expressing that we care for ourselves. We need fuel to function and putting premium fuel in the body improves overall performance. We try to eat living foods, fruits and vegetables closest to their natural state, to give us positive energy and a vast array of vitamins and minerals that cannot be duplicated by any supplement. We drink water daily to flush out the toxins and support cell processes. When we feel tired during the day or wake up tired after a good night's sleep, we might simply be a bit dehydrated—easily remedied with a cup of water. All our physical and mental processes depend on water.

Our bodies are designed to move. In most cultures prayer is associated with movement. When we exercise, we strengthen the skeletal frame to prevent osteopenia and osteoporosis in both men and women. Strength training will keep postures erect, shoulders back, feet firmly planted and our hearts open. The Surgeon General has predicted that by the year 2020 one out of two Americans will have osteoporosis. Exercising has been proven to help prevent this condition as well as prevent and treat cancer, type 2 diabetes, heart disease, depression and lessen the severity of many auto-immune diseases. Simply put, when we exercise, we get rid of stress hormones and increase our endorphins. We sleep better, eat better, and get fewer colds and infections. For a nation that looks to chemicals for relief from physical and psychic pain, exercise provides a healthier alternative. You decide: Prozac or Puma?

Although culturally we take pride in how little sleep we need, lack of sleep is unhealthy. During sleep the cells regenerate and heal. The mind heals by dreaming. Problems and conflicts trigger dreams the very same night and up to a week later where many of us suddenly find solutions to our difficult situations. People who get too little sleep experience memory problems, and the most serious driving accidents are not caused by drunken drivers, but by people who fall asleep at the wheel. When we begin the day with a sleep deficit, we are already irritable and anything can set us off, while the people around us absorb our increased stress levels. Insomnia ages the body and causes it to store fat around the middle.

While we can't control our natural environment—the air and the earth—we can be more vigilant about our home environment. We can try to avoid toxic chemicals and contaminated water, exposure to unnecessary radiation and to damp areas which harbor mold. It is easy enough not to microwave food wrapped in cling wrap which leaches toxins into foods; use a paper towel instead. Or if new carpeting is installed and wood floors are polyurethaned, we need to air out the room for a few days in order that the noxious chemicals can dissipate.

Rita learned that lesson after seeing many doctors. A group leader for Parkinson's patients and a part-time actress/song writer, Rita began to feel unnaturally exhausted and quiet. She felt so out of it that she had to write everything down because her memory was quickly fading. Sometimes she had difficulty breathing. Her job was in jeopardy from taking too many sick days. At first doctors told her it was all in her head and suggested that she see a psychiatrist. However, she didn't give up investigating because she felt the problem was in her body. One physician suggested that she see an allergist. After allergy testing, the results were in: she was off the charts for mold. When the doctor questioned her about where she lived, she explained that she had rented a walk-in apartment which had been recently renovated because of black mold. "Did you ever open a window?" "No, because I felt so sick and cold, I just lay in bed. I could barely move." "Rita, the more you stayed in a room with closed windows and without circulating air, the sicker you were getting by inhaling the black mold that I believe is still in the room! Renovations are more complicated when there is black mold. People can't simply cover it up with sheetrock—it will seep through. Ironically, all you had to do to feel better was to get up and get out! You sealed yourself in!"

To counteract unknown toxins in your environment bring fresh air and sunlight into your home. Grow house plants, like spider plants, Gerber Daisy, Dracaena Marginata, Peace lily (Spathiphyllum), Bamboo Palm, English Ivy and Chinese Evergreen, known to absorb harmful toxins and purify the air. An added benefit: green is the color of healing.

The emotional room

The emotional room of the house is more dramatic than the physical. When we enter this room, we stop over-thinking and over-analyzing. Instead this is where we cultivate our intuition: to get out of our minds and into our senses.

The byproduct of a mind which dissects everything is the inability to concentrate and accomplish. We feel tired during the day exhausted by our thoughts, yet at night, unable to rest, we lie in bed with eyes wide open counting our problems like sheep. The way to break this worry cycle is to stop trying to rationalize every experience with logical explanations and instead feel our way around our world with our senses.

The first step is to change our vocabulary from "I think" to "I feel." How do I feel about doing something or being with someone, as opposed to what I think I should do? To openly express our genuine feelings and act on them is liberating. Yet, saying the words, "I feel" is still a verbal expression of the rational mind. Human beings have the capacity to rationalize and justify anything. To truly get further into our feelings we can practice responding to our gut reactions. Animals are the first to sense an oncoming storm—way ahead of the meteorologists. When the Tsunami hit Indonesia, approximately three hundred thousand people perished. Strangely, none of the animals did. Some villagers recalled hearing shrieking birds and instinctually ran to higher ground for safety. Our animal natures are more honest and direct than our thoughts.

This does not mean that we should become vain or hedonistic and seek a life of carefree sensual pleasures. In order to satisfy head and heart, body and soul, we need to train the mind and body to work together in synchrony. If we are always in our head, we do not notice that our bodies are trying to tell us something; we lose our vitality and spontaneity, and increase the likelihood of disease or a breakdown in our relationships. We suppress our emotions and forget how to express our inner child. Here are some suggestions to get out of our heads and into our hearts:

Lose your mind

♦ Train yourself to be immersed in whatever you are doing. If you are distracted, empty your mind and clean out the clutter. Connect to what you are doing wholeheartedly.

♦ Sit still, breathe to your own natural rhythm; close your eyes for five minutes as you recall a palpable, joyous image or affirmation you memorized; look at a beautiful picture and close your eyes to experience it. Then begin your next activity.

♦ Focus on your breathing and visualize. Inhale a white fog, two counts through the nose and exhale a dark fog, four counts through the nose. With each breath feel your heart relaxing, beating to its natural rhythm.

♦ Pray to a Divine force as though you are opening your heart to a friend who loves you and accepts you just the way you are.

♦ Lose yourself in a good book or movie, which explores a theme, situation or relationship that parallels your life. A movie can help release suppressed feelings.

♦ Now that your mind is emptying, your senses become more alive. Experience your sense of smell, taste, touch, sound and sight. Feel the signals they send you. When you think about a specific person or situation and experience a bad smell or foul taste in your mouth, your primal intuition is trying to tell you something. Tap into it to avoid a painful event.

♦ If you are feeling anxious, where are you going or where have you just come from? To what or whom are your senses trying to direct your attention?

♦ If you experience a pain in you body, what is your body trying to tell you about your spirit? Ask yourself where in your body the pain has lodged and what it symbolizes: Is it your knees? A fear of moving forward. Your heart? Grief. Your back? Lack of support.

To be in touch with our emotions the goal is to live in the moment without worrying about the past or the future. That's where our minds wander in judgment. True, some moments are painful and sad. But they are only moments. Other moments are comical, loving and joyous. For example, a pregnant woman might throw up all morning feeling thoroughly sick. Yet in the evening she feels fine enjoying a delicious big meal. Whatever we are experiencing in life is temporary. We get overloaded and then like our muscles we adapt. Funny, how when we reflect on our past struggles, we remember the good old days. Let's vow to recognize and appreciate the good old days now!

The intellectual room

The intellectual room is brightly lit, for it is the reading room of the house. However, we learn not only by reading books, but also by reading life; we learn by listening to what others say—whether we agree or not. Controversy wakes us up. Daily we can stimulate the mind by learning something new, even if it is a vocabulary word, quote, or telephone number.

Often we get used to playing the role of always being right and giving advice. If we are more interested in speaking than listening, it is a sure symptom that we have become know-it-alls. We feel that we must speak to persuade others to our point of view. Perhaps, we don't have enough self-confidence, so we need to assert our truth over other people's voices. However, there is great power in listening.

I learned a great deal recently from a young woman just starting out as an intern in a highly competitive corporate law firm. She had to distinguish herself among the others in order to be asked to stay on when she graduated law school. There was cut-throat competition among interns, especially during meetings where the interns would make it a point to say anything at all just to be heard. Interactions on the TV show, *The Apprentice*, were tame by comparison. However, this young woman made up her mind to learn all that she could and speak only if she had something meaningful to say. She focused her interaction not with the partners of the firm, but with the junior lawyers of the pyramid. If she made mistakes, better with them, than with the partners. She learned from them and worked diligently and wholeheartedly for them. The junior lawyers were pleased and introduced her to the middle tier. She attended meetings and learned new skills. She worked methodically for long hours. Eventually, her name was brought up at a partners' meeting. She continued to focus on her work, listening and learning. Ultimately, she was invited to work directly for the partners while the other interns looked on in amazement.

We don't always need to go to school or read books to learn and grow intellectually. A great deal of learning occurs on the job like an apprentice. However, a crucial part of our education happens randomly from a word or two someone casually says in passing, or from a visual cue of a poster at the train station. When we visit the intellectual room of the house, our minds remain alert to these messages. Just three words can change a life.

Three words changed my life. After my father passed away from Alzheimer's, I missed him terribly, but I still had my mother and I was grateful. She was a sturdy, strong woman and I believed that we were free and clear of tragedy, somehow supernaturally protected from it by my father's death. However, two years later, she was also diagnosed with Alzheimer's. Lightening struck my household twice. When I told my friend about my mother's diagnosis, he simply said, "Debbie, lower your expectations." The minute I heard those words, I got it. My heavy heart felt so much lighter. For me this cryptic remark completely transformed my attitude. I smiled not a superficial, easy smile, but I smiled deep within. I realized that I still had my mother, for our relationship was still intact despite the disease. I made up mind to be thankful for each day and to take Kodak moments in my head of the good times— and there were many.

The spiritual room

The fourth room of the house is the spiritual. This room doesn't have to be found in a house of worship. Religion and spirituality as Anthony De Mello writes are sometimes polar opposites. I visit this room when I act kindly to other people. The spiritual room is actually a two-story room with a spiral staircase. On the first level, the main room, I *feel* compassionate toward other people and that's an important level to be on because we open our hearts to others, instead of living a closed, self-centered existence. We grow expansive. On the second story, the higher level, I *act* compassionately toward other people by concretely doing things for them. This higher level makes me feel happier and more self-confident because I give, no matter what my situation is.

Sometimes we lose touch with our own spirituality when bad things happen to us. We ask why me? It helps to accept what has happened without judgment because how do you accuse or judge a bacterium or virus, a car accident or a mudslide? Although we cannot restore or fix the world, we learn something about ourselves and others from how we respond to a disaster in order to move forward. We become more connected to each other through our vulnerability and when we are at peace with ourselves, there is at least some peace in the world.

Spiritual opportunities

Here are some suggestions to activate your spirituality:

- ◆ **Synchronize with nature and its energy.** This means slow down and ease on down the road. Absorb the beauty and train your eyes to observe the changes and the little inhabitants. Listen to the sounds of the wind, the birds, the rain and the leaves. Guess what? You are meditating!

- ◆ **Leave your head and get into your heart.** Trust your feelings more than your logical analysis. Your mind can play tricks on you.

- ◆ **Be receptive to revelations** in the simple words that are said to you, what you dream about, or what your eye is drawn to. Decode the clues.

- **Develop your five senses** to reach your sixth. Believe in your intuition and act on it. Don't override and dismiss your instinct.

- **See the ordinary with extraordinary eyes** as though you are seeing it for the first time experiencing your original delight.

- **Discover your creativity** and implement it. Act on what fills the ache in your heart and makes it sing. Delight in your self-expression and show it to the world. Act like a creator.

- **See the humor** inherent even in dark situations and conflicts. Laugh to release your inner light, realizing that suffering can make you a better person; adversity introduces you to a hidden part of yourself. Find the way out, the open door. By the way it's right next to that closed dark one!

- **Enjoy helping others,** saying a kind word to brighten someone's day and smiling when you make eye contact. Instead of complaining about the bad things people do or say, try complimenting the good things to generate good energy.

- **Cut others some slack.** Cultivate empathy and compassion. Everyone has an ego and wants to be right. Don't erode someone's ego and shame that person.

- **Heighten the connection between mind and body** through exercise and healthy eating. Living foods make you feel more alive. Remember to an important degree: you are what you eat.

- **Don't beat yourself up with guilt or regret.** Let go of your worries. Redirect your awareness to what makes you happy.

- **Create quiet time and space for yourself.** Believe that you are worth it!

When we visit all four rooms of the house daily, we pay attention to the structure, open the blinds, making it sunlit and warm. We develop an appreciation for the house we were freely given—a home that we did not have to earn: No complaints about what is missing—after all it is a gift. Comparisons to other houses do not make sense because each one is completely different, one of a kind. However, when I let my house fall apart because I do not value it enough to maintain it, then I deny a gift and a blessing. That weakens my spirit and my happiness.

We all know how the neighbors sneak a peek into each other's houses, peering through the slats of the blinds or looking out from the darkness into well-lit window views; it is important for our homes to be in order as anyone can be watching. Similarly, posture and energy convey a great deal about what is happening in our interior. If I slouch or trudge around, then I transmit negative vibes of depression to those I meet. If I walk slowly or hesitantly, perhaps, I am unsure and unsteady about what I have to do. If I run around, always huffing and puffing about how incredibly busy I am, then I am distracting myself from facing whatever I have to face. Maybe it's time for a house-cleaning!

A great thing about my house is that is has a sturdy front door with a double lock. I need not admit anyone negative. Because when I allow negativity to enter, the visits become more regular and I develop a tolerance and become desensitized to it. I begin to experience self-doubt and fatigue; I compromise my own relaxation time to take care of drama queens who become parasitic and more demanding. However, when my house is in order and all entry ways have protective locks, I need not admit any disturbing thoughts to my happiness or anyone who tries to undermine my positivism and discourage my enthusiasm.

When our houses are secure, we can withstand a tornado. Dorothy in the *Wizard of Oz* learned that there is no place like home. Home is where you are—in your heart.

- ◆ What kind of house do you live in?
- ◆ How many levels does it have including a basement and an attic?
- ◆ What is the condition of your house?
- ◆ Do you have enough space or do you feel confined?
- ◆ Do you visit all four rooms of your home everyday or do you tend to hang out in one room?

Now you might say, "That's cute, nice verbal play, but a little too glib. Have you considered the harsh effects of old age on our *homes*, despite the constant maintenance and care?" The elements and the seasons do their work. All we can do is to be the best that we can be as our homes age. While we can take refuge in our homes, we should not be *confined* or *defined* by them. The body is a repository for the soul. Our home is a gift—remember? We do not possess it.

During a stress-management workshop I gave for the *Woman's Network* one of the participants stood up and delivered a beautiful tribute to her mother who had died the previous year. Chris said, "My mother was a source of light to family and friends. In her eighties she became blind from macular degeneration and was crippled by painful arthritis. Yet she was cheerful, optimistic and loving. She was one of those people everyone wanted to be around because she was so interested in what you had to say. Every day was a good day for her and she never complained. I have to admit that I was amazed by her." I promised Chris that I would pay this story forward as a tribute to the golden light within us that never fades. Perhaps, this is why old age is referred to as the golden years. When *you prepare to die, you learn how to live.* All that is alive in the world becomes more precious to you. You begin again in the end. In fact, a universal ability is that we can begin again at anytime in our lives.

Similar to the four rooms in our house, there are four stages in our lives that parallel the birth process, or should I say, rebirth process. We experience all these stages, some more often than others. The good news is that no stage lasts forever because we give birth to ourselves many times during our lives.

Stage One

In the womb—the adult counterpart is just floating aimlessly through life, waiting, collecting information and energy, growing and trying to find out: who am I?

Stage Two

The head is engaged in the birth canal—the adult equivalent is being stuck, unable to act, fearing the unknown; there is no room to breathe or feel.

Stage Three

Breaking out, wailing—the adult equivalent is righteous anger, indignation, pressure, submission, pain, transformation, leading to the end of a stage.

Stage Four

Rebirth—the adult counterpart is creativity, liberation, inspiration, individuality, continued growth and empowerment.

Which stage describes your life at present? Are you just hanging out, stuck or angry? Perhaps you are ready to emerge into the light to breathe freely and on your own terms to experience what life presents. When you think about each stage, you see how each one is a necessary precursor to the next. All the stages are vital for personal growth and development.

Self-care Mantras

♦ The best kept beauty secret is health and vitality.

♦ Take Kodak moments in your head of the good times.

♦ Leave your head and get into your heart.

♦ We give birth to ourselves many times during our lives.

♦ See the ordinary with extraordinary eyes.

Chapter 7

THE DIFFERENCE BETWEEN PASSION AND COMPULSION

When we are preparing to seek employment, we need to distinguish a job from a career. A job is what we get paid to do. A career is about finding our authentic calling. When we discover whatever it is we love to do, we feel passion for our work. We are inspired and using our unique talents. Sometimes we lose track of time, and it appears to others that we have become workaholics because we are immersed in our work instead of interacting with them. When work transforms into fun and we balance it with a healthy personal life, we become successful in business, at home and with relationships.

Let's distinguish a passion for work from a compulsion for work which stems from neediness and insecurity—the constant need for validation. If our total identity is tied into our work, then we are running away from something. If we lose our jobs, do we lose ourselves? Ironically, many of the compulsive hours we spend at work don't accomplish the task we set out to do because we procrastinate our way to perfectionism; since nothing is ever perfect, we can never complete the project.

To find a career path that meets our passion for work, we need to be in touch with our emotions. It is like the Zen saying, "Your work is to discover your work, and then with all your heart to give yourself to it." When we do the work we love either at home or outside the home, we cultivate a sense of well-being and all our other relationships fall into place. Remember the old Disney song from *Snow White*, "Whistle while you work?" There is great wisdom in the lyrics. Here's an excerpt:

> Just whistle while you work
> Put on that grin and start right in
> To whistle loud and long
> Just hum a merry tune
> Just do your best and take a rest
> And sing yourself a song
>
> And as you sweep the room
> Imagine that the broom
> Is someone that you love
> And soon you'll find you're dancing to the tune
> When hearts are high the time will fly
> So whistle while you work.

Music and lyrics influence the rhythm of life. When you sing a happy song, you stimulate your neural machinery to elevate your mood. Rhythm is created by your routines. This song suggests that you find your rhythm both at home and at work.

Finding the right career

Finding the career for which we are best suited involves getting our personal needs met. As discussed in earlier chapters, many women block their path in life because everyone's needs always come first. We adjust to this pattern at a great personal cost! If we are unhappy, tired, irritable and work like a robot, it is time to find our true calling in life. It is never too late! Even if the people in our lives are shocked by this new emerging self, calling us selfish and chipping away at our self-confidence, it is only a challenge to awaken our personal determination from its slumber. Through educational training, networking and interning (even without pay) we will learn to love what we are doing and get paid for it besides.

To follow through on our passion and make a career move we first have to believe in ourselves. If we compare ourselves to other people, we sabotage our unique talents and abilities.

We might be telling ourselves that we are too old, too young, too poor, too uneducated, over-qualified, under-qualified, unlucky, too good, or not good enough.

To stop this negative self-talk: Make a list of your five best strengths and your five most important values. Get to know yourself better. Then connect with other people who share your values and your passion. You can do this through volunteer work or working as an intern without pay. You will learn a great deal in either scenario (consider it a free education) and will receive a solid letter of recommendation for a job well done. Interestingly enough, you will now have job experience without having worked in a formal job.

How to find your passion

In order to find your passion in your work objectively review your plusses and minuses. Make a list of your present capabilities as well as what used to make your heart sing—what ideas and hobbies you were once passionate about; think as far back as your childhood. The next step is not to be in awe of other people. They are just fellow human beings. Face the fears of uncertainty, rejection and failure that are holding you back. Most of them are fueled by your imagination. If you have not had a good run at work lately, recall your past successes and what personal traits helped you. Now recall these good qualities to life and transfer them to daily living to achieve health and happiness. Then use them in a new line of work you will enjoy. Apply your innate gifts to the real world. For example, if you are persuasive and people respond to you, then you might choose a career such as a teacher, actor, attorney, politician or salesperson. There are many possibilities; be alert to recognizing opportunities. They won't come knocking at your door; you have to find them. In the last step, let your mind wander and imagine a full day working in a career that you love.

A point to remember when beginning or changing your job: it might be part of a natural cycle of change for you. And you might change again and again throughout the years. I have been an English teacher, a writer, a stress-management specialist and now I am a radio show host and a writer. I was passionate about each phase and then reinvented myself into the next one when my heart told me to move on. Change felt natural and necessary like shedding old skin to reveal what is new and fresh underneath. An intense feeling urged me to try something new. Trust your inner urgings!

How to let work, work for you

Sister Loyola Curtin directs outreach programs at her parish like the CEO of a corporation. "God is in management and all of us are in sales and service. We all have our gifts and talents and God is cognizant of them. He needs different personalities."

In her 70s, Sr. Loyola still walks with a spring in her step, going up and down the stairs and rushing down the long corridors. She is feisty and passionate about her outreach programs. Whenever necessary, she rolls up her shirt sleeves and gets to work packaging food and flowers for the shut-ins. Sister Loyola revealed what she learned: "When I first started out, I thought I would save the world. I soon realized that I was called forth to set programs in motion and then to step aside. I help people discover what they can do to help themselves. It's called empowerment. Simplicity works for me. I present the program for the incoming group and I give up control a few weeks later when they are running it and feel connected to one another. I spend time observing the groups, especially the leadership and then disappear, returning every so often to see how things are going. When you aren't using your energy to control, you don't get used up! There is absolutely no need to get tired. You can keep on creating by delegating."

Part of Sister Loyola's success is due to her flexibility and creativity. Her mind is forever young with an unusual capacity for growth and change. "We have to allow people to find their own way of serving. People are not called to the same things in the same way. There is new life in a new way." And by the way no one calls her Sister which she perceives as an artificial label. "It divides us into clerical and non-clerical. If I'm religious, are you non-religious?"

Workaholics

Unlike creative passion, you realize that you have become compulsive at work when your life is out of balance. This is obvious when you are spending less and less time at home interacting with the family. Even if you are a homemaker and caregiver, you might be investing more into cleaning, cooking and PTA than in time with the family. Just because you are at home or work at home, doesn't mean that you are really there. You might be going through the motions of a daily routine while tuning everyone out.

Attending a school event or visiting elderly parents while you conduct business on your cell phone means that you are really *not* present for your loved ones. Similarly, if you worry about your family while you are at work, you don't do your work wholeheartedly. Because of technology like computers and cell phones, we can work 24/7 anywhere. Therefore it is getting increasingly difficult to establish balance in our lives, separating work from home. Many of us have created work-stations in the bedroom and then wonder why we have trouble sleeping. When our lives are out of balance, it could be that you are running away from a deep-rooted unhappiness, or suppressing a crisis and keeping busy helps you to keep your mind off your problems.

Workaholism—an official addiction

Workaholism—deemed an official addiction by the American Medical Association—destroys lives. Whether you sense that you are becoming a workaholic or your family and co-workers are telling you that you are one, it's time to break the cycle and establish more regular hours.

Most workaholics need to be working constantly in order to feel like they have some semblance of control, structure and validation, and so they seek out jobs that allow them to exercise their addictions.   They work at high-stress jobs to keep the adrenaline rush going. Workaholics take their parenting so seriously that there is no balance in their lives—no hobbies, fun or spirituality. All their time is with the PTA, scouts and the soccer team.

Workaholics tend to be products of demanding parents who expect huge accomplishments from their kids. These children grow up always seeking their parents' approval—alive or dead. Because perfection is unattainable, workaholics will always try harder, strive to be better. There is never an end or a completion to a project.

Workaholics tend to be less effective than other employees because they're not team players. They are usually suspicious believing that their co-workers will take credit for their work. They have trouble delegating work, sharing information and take too much upon themselves. On paper they look good and corporations encourage them, but this compulsiveness regarding work comes at a personal cost to health and relationships.

A tale of two homes

Nellie, one of the young professional mothers participating in my stress-management workshop for establishing work-home balance, decided that she had to change her perception of home. Because she worked at home and was available to her daughters and did not have to commute to an office, she had the best of both worlds. She took pride as a feminist who earned her keep and had a housekeeper to do the traditionally feminine duties. She and her husband owned two homes and Nellie worked hard in her city home to pay for her summer home in Vermont. Her city home duplicated a corporate work environment—a constant reminder of the work at hand. The summer home was more like a traditional home serving as a quiet retreat: no computers or fax machines. When I suggested that she had lost a sense of home in her primary dwelling, she laughed until the tears rolled down her cheeks.

Nellie decided to set up some work/home boundaries. No more working late into the night and this is a big one—*scheduled* family dinners, prepared with her pre-teen daughters. She realized that a bit of domesticity helped create warmth and closeness and did not detract from her independence, rather it rounded her out as a person. Perhaps, the lady had protested too much after all.

During the family dinner ritual she invited her young daughters to contribute their opinions to the adult discussion which made them feel important. Nellie and her husband discovered that they enjoyed each other's company and that they had two terrific daughters who were quite intelligent. As a result, the girls performed much better at school going from average grades to A's. Nellie accomplished even more at work as she eased up on her schedule. She found that she had fresh energy and greater creativity because of her work/home balance. Her new work ethic: *if it doesn't get done today, it will get done the next, or the day after.*

Many women who leave their intense careers to become stay-at-home-moms feel as though they are missing something. The most obvious loss is that much-needed second income. The more subtle loss is a fulfilling and meaningful work identity. This is not to say that being a caregiver to children, elderly parents or a spouse is not meaningful; however, the many stay-at-home-moms I meet in the course of my sessions are searching for personal creative fulfillment. To put it bluntly women are searching for a future not defined by *should,* but rather by *could* or *would.*

You go, girl!

The good girl syndrome is hard to give up as it is ingrained in our psyche. "Now go ahead and be a good little girl, won't you?" Most of us have heard this from our mothers (who were also encouraged to be good little girls) and from our fathers who expected it from their wives and their daughters. Every girl grows up basking or wishing to bask in the sunlight of her father. If a father doesn't tell a daughter that she is special, doesn't encourage her, or make her feel better when she fails, she will have low self-esteem unless her mother can compensate for the loss. That is why so many women strive to find their passion outside themselves.

There is a mighty struggle that occurs in the heart of every woman. She feels stressed by the disparity between what she wants to do and what she feels she has to do. In Victorian times they called this vague unhappiness, the *vapors.* Freud called it *hysteria.*

Creativity begins at home

At some point in every woman's life she must set out on a creative journey of self-fulfillment. It can begin by opening all your senses to what stimulates you. Creative energy is all around you. Take mental note of it and assimilate it. The inspiration will dissipate and vanish unless your implement it.

Beth was always interested in both art and computers, but she forgot about it while she was raising her family. Even with her two children attending high school full time, she was feeling more tired than ever. During one of my stress-management sessions a member of the support group diagnosed Beth's problem, "You feel so tired because you are bored. What do you really enjoy doing?" Beth didn't know. I advised her to give it some thought and to be on the lookout. A few days later flipping through a neighborhood flyer, Beth noticed an adult education course schedule. The course in Computer Graphics attracted her attention and the time frame was perfect. She loved both the subject and the teacher and the following semester took a more advanced class. She began experimenting on her computer and learning new programs. Beth is off to a good start in her new career—designing brochures and logos for businesses, invitations and tee shirts. Although Beth no longer attends my stress-management group, she let us know that she is no longer tired!

When you are in the process of developing your creativity, part of it will be ego driven. By taking guidance and exchanging ideas with similar creative minds, you will be receptive to more signs. Also, you will be able to release all that self-imposed pressure by easing up on yourself. Giving up single-minded control will help unblock and release your inspiration.

When you are ready to implement your ideas, carve out a specific time and space at home. Let your friends and family know that although you are physically at home, you are really working! This will take some time to convey to others and for them to absorb. Your friends will ring your doorbell or call to socialize and the school will ask you to serve pizza at lunch because "you are a stay-at-home-mom." You will have to work hard to establish your work/home boundaries. Keep your phone machine on to screen phone calls, and don't forget to pull down the blinds, so the nosy neighbors and friends don't peek in and say, "Oh, you're home!"

One of the greatest benefits of tapping into your creative energy is that it will cheer you up and make you feel more alive. When you feel an empty ache in your heart, or feel alienated from other people because of illness or loss, creativity will counteract the destructive forces by filling you with joy and purpose.

This true story touched my heart and stirred those in my workshop. A woman in her early 60s suffered a severe stroke which left her paralyzed on the right side of her body. She had to be moved to a nursing home in order that her special needs could be met. Having to live among nursing home patients depressed her since she had been a rather active woman. A few months later she began to participate in art therapy classes held at the nursing home. Intuitively, she realized that painting might cheer her up and would provide a whole new experience. She told the instructor that she couldn't paint because she had lost the use of her right hand. "What about your left hand?" Reluctantly, she picked up a paint brush. She blossomed through her art. Her work was exhibited in one show and then many others followed. Her paintings sold easily. She confessed that she never would have taken up painting if she did not have a stroke! Adversity can challenge us to explore a different route to creativity and self-growth. In this case the evidence is remarkably tangible.

Ultimately, the difference between passion and compulsion is the difference between positive and negative energy. The most essential question to ask yourself: Are you at peace with yourself? The answer to this question will help you to know the difference.

Self-care Mantras

♦ When you aren't using your energy to control, you don't get used up.

♦ When you feel an empty ache in your heart, creativity will fill you with joy and purpose.

♦ Change feels natural and necessary like shedding old skin to reveal what is new and fresh underneath.

♦ If it doesn't get done today, it will get done the next, or the day after.

♦ Search for a future not defined by should, but rather by could or would.

Chapter 8

DON'T BURN OUT, REVITALIZE

"Everyday can't be Christmas, Debbie. We just wouldn't appreciate it if we were celebrating everyday!" Carla said during my workshop on how to have fun. Loosely translated, "Debbie, you just sound too slick about happiness." Another participant seconded the motion: "Yes, I quite agree with Carla. The celebration of a holiday or special occasion needs the build-up of anticipation. That is the real joy." Carla added, "Besides, my children don't even value the presents anymore. They have too much and the holidays have lost most of their spiritual context."

Everyone was getting stirred up and rebellious about the holidays. Happiness was fast becoming an illusion as the discussion took a detour into the weekday routine. Betty chimed in about hating to have to get up every morning to work at a job that she found boring. Wendy added that she needed to leave her job because she resented being used, but felt guilty about leaving the people who depended on her. "Wait a minute, everyone. I don't mean to gloss over your issues, but all this negativity has a purpose. Adversity introduces you to yourself. If you can view yourself objectively and truthfully regarding your strengths and limitations, then great joy is coming to you. Contrast helps us to define and appreciate who we are and what we can do. If you can accept your truth along with other people's truths, you can ease up on life instead of beating your head against a wall. Instead of anticipating holiday joy a month beforehand, why can't we anticipate daily joy? Time is relative and subjective. If you like what you are doing, time flies. If you don't like what you are doing, time is endless. The answer is obvious: love what you are doing and if you don't, change it, so that you do. Wake up every morning and anticipate what a fun day it will be. Fulfill your own psychic prediction—prove yourself right."

There is a purpose to venting when we feel hurt, frustrated, angry or sad. However, the goal is not just to scream or cry for its own emotional sake. Venting is what happens on the way to self-discovery. Venting stimulates us to release suppressed emotions, process them and finally recognize the truth about ourselves and the situation. Now we are ready to **reinvent**!

No job is too small

One of the most common reasons for burnout is the complaint that the job has become too small. However, no job is too small for you; sometimes you are too small for the job. You need to reinvent your job. Imagine this scenario. You can't get a job in your field right now because the market is tight. You compromise and take a job at the post office. It is steady work and gives you good benefits. However, you have a Masters degree in genetic research and begin to feel that it is beneath you to stamp envelopes, weigh packages and issue money orders; after all you should be working with gene mapping instead of zip code maps. Suddenly, you observe your colleague working alongside you. He smiles at everyone and asks familiar customers how they are feeling and what is new in their lives. He asks an elderly woman how her daughter's surgery went and she says, "That is so kind of you. I woke up feeling sad and worried about her. But your concern shows me that somebody out there cares. I feel so much better. You don't know how much you have brightened my day!"

Our friend, the DNA researcher, experienced a slightly humbling epiphany that he was too small for the job. On the other hand, his colleague touched so many people in a good way that it was impossible to quantify the rippling effect of his kind words and good energy. He had found a way to make the mundane extraordinary. If this were a movie, his colleague would be an angel disguised as a postal worker. The truth is that we can all be angels in disguise. We don't have to save the world, but we can cheer up and help people in small things that matter greatly. Emily Dickinson wrote: *A word said is never dead.*

A disgruntled attitude stems from a perceived lack of empowerment. The DNA researcher who couldn't get a job in his chosen academic field, internalized the failure and felt as though he wasn't good enough. His response at the post office was to compensate for his self-imposed inadequacy with "I'm too good to be here." If you have a fundamental appreciation for who you are and what you have learned in life, then a seemingly menial task cannot possibly trivialize you.

During World War II my mother cleaned stables on a Polish farm while she was hiding from the Nazis. She didn't feel demeaned by her work. Instead she felt blessed to be alive and privileged to be able to clean horse manure in a stable, instead of experiencing starvation, humiliation and ultimately death in a concentration camp. You see, everything boils down to perception. My mother always had a strong sense of who she was and what she could do. A menial job or an insulting word could not diminish her spirit. She didn't let the negativity penetrate her. Working as a slave on a farm saved her life. There were millions who were less fortunate.

Anything routine can be infused with creativity, fun or freshness—if you change your traditional-always-done-it-this-way perception. For example, Sister Claire at St. Gregory's in Bellerose, Queens has revitalized the droning repetition of chanting which is popular in Eastern meditation. I personally witnessed how she revivified the "Our Father." She is able to concentrate on each word because she lists by name all the foreign countries, cities, political leaders, friends, family members and the people she encounters who need a prayer said for them. Sister Claire will simply say, "Jesus, Iraq. Jesus, Southeast

Asia. Jesus, Israel. Jesus, Aunt Jill, Jesus . . ." Each time Sister Claire says the Lord's Prayer, she personalizes it with those who need God's attention at that time. The list varies daily; she has customized a general prayer with her intentions. Needless to say: it takes her a long time to get through her prayer!

Rearrange your furniture and rearrange your life

Similarly, if you are bored with your home, your furniture, your knick-knacks and your environment, you don't need to move away or do extensive renovations. Simply moving things around, rotating your collectibles to different shelves, tables or mantels makes them appear new. Hang your paintings on other walls and see them with the same excitement of the first time. Modify their lighting because a different angle of light provides a new angle of perception. Change where you sit at the kitchen table or move your desk to a new part of the room and wake up your senses.

You know the expression: *location, location, location.* Dr. Bernie Siegel was always bothered by the way he sat behind a big desk which subtly transmitted to patients that he was the great all-knowing father while they were sitting in front of it, gazing into his eyes awaiting their life and death sentences. Emotionally, the huge mahogany desk served as a barrier—the vast difference in status between oncologist/surgeon and cancer patient. Bernie moved his desk against the wall and sat right next to his patients. He realized that his view had changed because he could now see with more empathic eyes the whole person he was treating.

Because we have a tremendous capacity to adapt, we tend to get bored with what we once enjoyed and treasured. Moreover, because we are programmed for spiritual growth, we need to evolve in our work and relationships in order to experience inner fulfillment. We don't usually like the same clothes, foods, TV shows and vacations that we did twenty years ago. If you reread a book you loved a decade ago, you will discover new ideas in it. If you don't see anything new, then I boldly assert that you have not grown as a person.

Put passion back into your chores

If you have fallen into a mild depression because your daily routine consists of one drudgery after another—the Cinderella complex—you need to revitalize your chores. Can you perform your tasks with alacrity, so that you get an exercise benefit from washing the floor, vacuuming, ironing, food shopping or bathing a loved one? Wouldn't it be wonderful to do housework and caregiving with a new consciousness—that you are getting a healthy aerobic/strength training workout while accomplishing it. When you lift that laundry basket, you are doing a deep squat. When you carry the laundry basket to the basement and back, you are lifting weights. When you vacuum quickly, you are raising your heart rate. When you bathe an elderly parent, you are maintaining her dignity and your own.

Can you play your favorite songs while you do your routine tasks? Wouldn't music lift your spirits and make you, as well as those you care for, just want to move, clap their hands or sing along? If you select music with a strong fast beat, you will feel your positive energy levels rising. Your happiness will be absorbed by your entire household, including the pet.

While doing mundane tasks, you can let your mind soar. Try composing poetry the next time you make the beds, or write a song as you mop the floor. While you automatically do the routine with your body, your mind can creatively visualize the specific goals and stages of a project—using that so-called meaningless time to develop something that makes you feel alive.

Above all, try not to see your work as futile and meaningless. See your chores as contributing to the aesthetics of the environment. We all have an innate love of beauty. By cleaning and shining up our setting, we create a spiritually and visually appealing place that welcomes others into our world. When our home is messy and cluttered, we close ourselves off, not letting anyone inside. The same applies to personal hygiene. Nobody loves changing a dirty diaper. However, when the baby or adult in your care, is fresh and clean, there is a sense of the purity and wholesomeness of the human form.

If you can't fix it, change it!

In life we have to stretch our energy to see how far we can expand and grow. Sometimes we outgrow our career and cannot reinvent it. I taught English literature for many years. I can't even count how many times Hamlet perished in my classroom or Oedipus blinded his eyes. Strangely, I was never bored; it always felt like the first time and I was easily moved to tears by the beautiful words. I perceived the perfection in human imperfection in these masterpieces. Also, bright student eyes fueled the appreciation; I listened to the analysis of open minds eager to invent something new about Shakespeare or Sophocles. Quite often a student made an interesting and profound comment and I learned a new idea or new perspective I had never considered before.

After twenty years of teaching, however, I was feeling a little burned out with the career context, not with the students or the material. The signs were there. Each morning I was beginning to feel less eager to go to work. I returned home exhausted. The paycheck, benefits and pension were not enough to keep me there. I could have relied on the same notes to coast through my classes, assigning fewer research papers and giving multiple choice exams to make the job easier and more palatable. Instead, at the height of my game, I left after giving proper notice. I believe that we should always do things correctly, especially when we choose to leave a job, because that is how we will be remembered. Consequently, I gave up a highly structured environment and a well-respected identity to start a new career without a title, track record or network. It felt like a free fall, yet it also felt exciting like a wonderful adventure. I recovered a sense of joy. I gave birth to myself again!

Come from the heart

Whatever you do needs to come from the heart and do it wholeheartedly! In order to love your work, you have to know how to love in the first place. Love demands a lot from you and sometimes you get tired of your work and your environment. However, that overall feeling of love for your work keeps you there and overrides the boredom of all the routine tasks every career, household and relationship entail.

Any work that you do emanates from you, the control center. What or who could be more fascinating and special than you? When you shift your attitude to appreciating your work, affirming it and putting your imagination into it, you can recreate your job. Don't expect your boss to recreate your job. Your boss runs a department and must answer to her supervisors. When anyone in the group makes a mistake, the boss assumes responsibility for it. Also, she has to sustain a vision for the entire team. Therefore the boss does not have the time or the same energy as you do, to devote to your projects. Here's what you can do to transform your work experience:

- ◆ Approach your work from a different angle.
- ◆ Stick to the moment at hand. Don't think about future acknowledgment, a change in management or monetary compensation. Do your work with integrity and the rest will follow.
- ◆ Talk to people in your field and network your way to new ideas.
- ◆ Take classes to learn new things about your work. You will feel more confident about suggesting new projects.

♦ Invest your project with time. You can come to work earlier and leave work a bit later occasionally.

♦ Be available for questions and share your knowledge. Soon everyone will know that you are the expert to consult on this subject. If you focus long enough on a small area, you will become the specialist and it is easier to become an authority on a specific topic.

Plan on retiring? Forget about it!

I have noticed a trend among women regarding retirement. In the past women eagerly anticipated traveling, doing less housework as the nest emptied out, resuming hobbies after a long career and mainly easing on down the road. Nowadays many women plan on working longer and put off retirement. My close friend, Susan, sees these years as the most stimulating of her life as she manages a billion dollar fund. She has knowledge, wisdom, ambition, curiosity and energy. She built her career from the bottom up starting as an administrative assistant. Susan learned to re-create her work. She became an acknowledged expert on small cap stocks and then moved on to the next phase of her development. Currently, her children are off to college and on their own. She can channel her energy and focus on new arenas. She loves networking with highly charged out-of-the-box people because they stimulate her. In contrast, she has observed the men in her field looking for peace and quiet after many years on Wall Street, "Female executives are just coming into their own in their fifties. It's their turn to shine. In a complete reversal, high-powered male executives are content to stay at home, take care of the children and run the household. It's like the changing of the guard."

A number of seniors in my "Silver Sneakers" program related that within two years of their retirement, they found that they couldn't handle all the free time, and they experienced a loss of identity and a lack of respect. They emphasized that they needed more stimulation; after traveling for awhile and playing with the grandchildren, they were bored. They missed feeling a sense of contribution and having a meaningful structure in their lives. Some chose to work part-time to have the best of both worlds. Some returned to school to update their skills in order to reenter the workforce or completely change careers. Ruth graduated from Brooklyn College with her grandson. They both majored in English and took many classes together. She earned a higher GPA than he did!

Those who found it difficult to get a job because of *unofficial* age discrimination did volunteer work. Others decided to write their memoirs. In these days of on-demand publishing one can leave a bound legacy to future generations. A wonderful byproduct of writing one's memoirs is sharpening the mind while looking back and saying, "Wow, did I accomplish all this?"

The bush burned, but was not consumed

No matter what your age is, or what you do, instead of burning out, burn up with passion. Take chances and choose wisely. Think of the Biblical archetype of Moses and the burning bush. The bush burned but was not consumed. God spoke to Moses through that fiery shrub. The spiritual message is that creativity sets us on fire, but does not consume us. Creative people notice what others don't see—unusual juxtapositions and inventive perceptions—they expect the unexpected—not necessarily inventing something completely new, never before seen. Moses was amazed by what he saw and listened to the message. He was receptive and absorbed the burning bush's powerful energy, potent enough to make him a leader. If we are not open to these signs, we will not see the miracles in our daily lives. If we do not connect with other people who share our passion, we will not learn important information that can help us to implement our vision.

I recommend the creative process if you are trying to lose weight. When I write, I am on fire. My metabolism speeds up. I am more energetic and joyous. Actually, people ask me if I am taking drugs to elevate my mood! Often I wake up in the middle of the night with an idea and am driven to write it the next morning. I do not write alone, for I know that I am a conduit through which past voices speak. Once the words are written, they take on an independent life, their own reality. I set them free.

Therefore if destructive things are happening in your life like illness or a career setback, don't be consumed by the struggle and the disappointment. Instead, reverse it with creation. Use the fiery process to burn off what is unnecessary to get to the essence. Free yourself from a self-destructive mindset. Create your reality and open your heart to love and fulfill yourself because it feels so good and the world needs what you can give it.

Self-care Mantras

- Wake up every morning and anticipate what a fun day it will be. Fulfill your own psychic prediction—prove yourself right.
- Don't vent; reinvent.
- Stretch your energy to see how far you can expand and grow.
- In order to love your work, you have to know how to love in the first place.
- Creativity will set you on fire; not consume you. Create your reality.

Chapter 9

MAKE THE HUMDRUM HOLY

We're always waiting for a milestone to be happy. It's the same old song for most people. I'll be happy **when** I: *graduate, get a job, get married, get some money, get divorced, when the kids grow up, retire . . .*We postpone living by fantasizing about the future. When it happens, we are still not satisfied. We ask: "Is this what I have been waiting for?" All this proves that happiness needs a sustained and continuous effort.

Somehow we grow accustomed to unhappy thoughts. Medical research studies focus on unhappiness rather than happiness! Why do we tolerate negativity in ourselves and those around us? It is acceptable, even expected of us to be mildly irritable while cheerfulness has become an anomaly. People quickly assume that we are utilizing feel-good chemistry if we smile a lot or move with energy; in other words we must be taking Paxil, Zoloft, or another drug.

We take an important step toward reinforcing our own positive thinking and get a quick high without side effects when we help others. Generously taking the time to tutor someone reinforces the material in your mind to learn it better. Even when you're sick or feel cornered by personal problems, you can feel better immediately when you serve others. On a palpable level you grasp that no matter how you feel, you still have power to make an important contribution. You move yourself from the narrow and isolating context of personal suffering which leaves you feeling lonely into the larger context of accomplishment and belonging.

No holy places and no holy people, only holy moments

Another direct route to happiness is focusing on the little things, sensing the details and appreciating them. We can delight in the obvious. Here's an example from my own back-yard. I was entertaining cousins who had just arrived from the hot climate of the Middle East. They were visiting here in autumn to experience its glory—something new for them. It was early October and since I lived on Long Island, not in New England, the leaves had not changed color yet. Our cousins had always been fascinated by the whole mysterious process of falling leaves, something I took for granted, or even felt annoyed about because I had to rake and bag them. In fact, our cousins were amateur photographers and intent on taking hundreds of shots to get that special photo. After a week of touring New York City, they rented a car and headed out to Vermont where it was peak season for autumn leaves.

Three weeks later, the leaves finally changed on Long Island. The vibrant colors surprised me, seemingly changed overnight. The following week on the way to Manhattan, I noticed that the wild, overgrown vines clinging to the newly-constructed concrete highway barriers were also in the process of changing color. I wondered why the same vines were in three different stages: green, gold and red. Perhaps it was the angle of the sunlight or maybe some of the leaves were younger than others. I speculated how our Israeli cousins would view these wild vines and what imaginative photos they would shoot. I began to study my environment with a tourist's eye. If I were a tourist abroad, I would surely appreciate every little rock or crack in the wall the guide pointed out to me.

Because we grow accustomed to our surroundings, our jobs, spouses, children, good health, friends, or basic comforts, we begin to feel bored and more prone to find fault, justifying the need for more exotic stimulation. Here is where the imagination can transform the commonplace into the astonishing. When I was living in Belle Harbor, New York, my next door neighbor Mary rented out her house for the summer to a couple from France while she and her husband and son traveled cross country. Although our homes had a similar layout, my home was filled with the sounds and clutter of two rambunctious boys dousing one another with water guns while laundry waited to be sorted, housecleaning finished and dinner prepared.

From my upstairs bedroom window which faced my backyard and Mary's, I spied unabashedly on the summer tenants. I was surprised to see that every evening on Mary's redwood table stood a white bud vase with a freshly picked rose from her garden adorned by two creamy linen place settings, ivory china and wine glasses. In their beach attire, sipping wine while delicately munching on cheese and crackers, the French couple gazed at the sunset, talking softly.

Are they crazy? I muttered under my breath. This is not a quaint vacation cottage, but Mary's regular clapboard three-bedroom house, just like many on our block. As soon as my husband walked in the house with the usual, "Isn't dinner ready yet?" I called him upstairs for a look out the window—a picture is worth a thousand words. "The French really know how to live," he laughed. The next day I set our redwood table with wine glasses and plates laden with snacks. My boys were still running around shooting their high-powered water guns, but my perspective had changed. I realized that my home could be a vacation resort, too. "Just look at that amazing sunset, Steve."

If we recognize what is before our eyes, then what is hidden will be revealed to us. We create our personal happiness. Chances are good that happiness already resides in our home. We just need to turn up the light to make it more visible. It reminds me of the children's picture book, *I Spy*. To spot the camouflaged object on the page we need to look at it from every angle. Once we spot it, we're surprised at how long it took to detect it in the first place and can always readily identify it thereafter.

Here are some tips to turn your days to breathless beauty:

♦ Take frequent walks in your neighborhood. Take note of sights, sounds, fragrances and textures. Bring your camera and photograph inspired compositions.

♦ If you have a hard time appreciating what is in your life, go the opposite route. Deprive yourself for a short time and then experience it again. You are more likely to appreciate a thing by missing it for awhile. You would never value vacation if you didn't work.

♦ Serve your meal with a beautiful presentation and chew your food slowly to savor taste and texture. Pretend you are leisurely dining at an inn.

♦ Read the *Book of Job* and you will find it easier to appreciate ordinary everyday things in your life.

Here is an anecdote to help us to appreciate the little things in life. During World War II a man was stranded on a raft in the middle of the ocean for twenty-one days. He survived with a modicum of food and water from rain and sea. A few months after his rescue, he was interviewed by the press, "What are you most happy about now that you have returned home? He answered, "Having enough food and water."

Medical science validates optimism

Seeing the glass as half-full rather than half empty may pay off in terms of a longer life. In a medical research study that spans more than a decade which evaluated men and women ages 65-85 regarding morale, self-respect and health, over 50% of the participants proved that optimism prolongs life. The reasons are:

♦ Optimism is associated with more physical activity, moderate alcohol use and less smoking.

♦ Optimism is associated with better health in general. People in poor health tend to be pessimistic.

♦ Optimists cope with stress more effectively than pessimists do.

To be optimistic rid yourself of limiting assumptions like: *I can't; It will never work; It's too difficult; I never did it this way before; They will think that I'm an idiot.* Instead befriend yourself and give yourself a pep talk. Fill yourself with good energy by going someplace where you feel happy and uplifted. It might be a house of worship, a museum, the beach, or a friend's house. Absorb the good energy of the place.

Sound and sense your way to optimism

The keys to happiness are old and stored inside you through memory and association. A fragrance or song can evoke a positive or negative association from the past and color your mood. For some of us, the aroma of vanilla is sweet and delightful and effective for managing stress; for another person the aroma of vanilla is nauseatingly sweet because it is connected with a difficult person or a demanding situation.

Similarly the lyrics to childhood songs might cheer you up and make you feel protected and loved, or they might hold painful and abusive associations. Reflect on what makes your own heart sing and inhale the personal aromas of happier times to give you a subliminal lift which will trigger your mind to supply the logical reason to reinforce your happiness. In this way the limbic brain works with the cognitive brain.

While I was writing this, serendipitously, I heard *Somewhere Over the Rainbow* from the radio. Immediately, my spirit began to soar as it revisited a more innocent time of childhood. I felt a deep down enjoyment, more hope regarding my work, an openness to new possibilities and a fundamental appreciation of my home—there's no place like it. Happiness resides within the self.

Often we miss opportunities in our lives because we are not fully present to what we are doing—that momentary experience of being truly alive. By opening ourselves up to experience fresh, new moments, we give ourselves over to our senses which help us to be in touch with what is really going on inside as well as outside us. We don't have to struggle and analyze. Here's how to easily find allusive happiness through our senses:

♦ *Feel* around your world. If you suddenly hear an old song, how does it make you feel? If you smell freshly baked bread, how does it make you feel? Our senses are more honest than our busy logical minds which play verbal tricks. If you feel sad, duplicate a sensual experience from a childhood song that still makes you happy and encourages you to laugh. **Sing it!** Don't just listen to it. What message does it contain? Act on it!

♦ If you need to slow down, drink a soothing hot liquid that makes you feel warm and relaxed inside like hot chocolate, herbal tea, coffee or soup. Because it is hot, it will permeate your body with warmth and you will have to drink it slowly to really taste and enjoy it.

♦ Practice becoming a psychic medium. Take note of your sense impressions to the various stimuli in your life. If you feel a tense knot in your stomach or a bad taste in your mouth when a person is talking to you, be aware of the physical relay system and move away from the negative energy. If your eyes are drawn to a word on a license plate or a billboard on the road, what is the message for you?

Fall in love again

Most importantly, if you want to awaken your optimism to the highest degree, then you must fall in love. Now you don't have to fall in love with a significant other, but you do have to fall in love. Your love might be for your children, your God, your home, your pet, your work, for nature, for education, for a political cause, or for your support group. Do you remember how you felt when you first fell in love, that everything was rosy and you virtually floated into rooms? You laughed at things other people didn't even think were funny. You believed in yourself and that life was filled with infinite possibilities. You had dreams and were determined to make them happen.

All right, I know that we are seasoned by adversity and a bit more cynical because we have interacted with other people's negative energy. When something bad and painful happens in our lives, many of us ask, "Why me? What did I do to deserve this? After all I am a good person and I prayed to God; why weren't my prayers answered?" These questions can inherently become more disturbing and more stressful than the original problem itself. We place a guilty load on our shoulders, lose trust in God and can't let go of feeling like a victim. In contrast we also swing on the emotional pendulum to the opposite extreme; we spend a great deal of time hoping. Although we need hope to create an optimistic trigger to help us to move forward, if we hope for the wrong things, we rob ourselves of accepting and then adapting to the present situation. Human beings are beautifully engineered to adjust. We can live with and work through our grief.

True story: A young, unmarried woman of thirty-three was diagnosed with breast cancer and needed a radical mastectomy. She resigned herself to never marrying because of her surgery. Her post-surgical treatment which included the full course of radiation treatment caused a common side effect, lymphedema, an uncomfortable swelling of her arm. She went for lymphedema massage therapy to deal with this uncomfortable side-effect. Not in her wildest dreams could she imagine the complete happy resolution of her illness. She and her massage therapist fell in love and are engaged to be married! Out of adversity sprouted true love!

In early February 2004 an Australian study, "Optimism and Survival in Lung Carcinoma Patients," stated that optimism in a group of patients with a specific type of cancer did not lengthen their lives. The conclusion: The role of optimism had been highly overrated in cancer survival. While this study undermined the role of positive thinking in healing, many physicians still continued to support the theory that positive thinking was effective in improving life quality. Dr. Abraham Verghese in a February 22, 2004 *NY Times* article explained that thinking we have supernatural, positive powers to drive away illness is simplistic. However, positive thinking helps us *to live with an illness* instead of *die from it*. Hope is a wonderful thing—Emily Dickinson called it, "The thing with feathers." However, we have to simplify our hope keeping it realistic and reasonable.

Don't be the judge who finds you guilty!

Many of us are highly experienced and extremely creative when it comes to conjuring up disturbing, guilt-ridden feelings. We start to feel sorry for ourselves, displeased, disappointed or just plain miserable. Here are some of the guilty thoughts that people have shared. Just saying them out loud in our group session prompted tears of relief and freedom. In fact, one guilty revelation prompted another, "If you didn't open up and say that you felt guilty, I never would have opened up either. I have never said this aloud to anyone." Here is a sampling of their deep-felt sharings:

- ◆ It's been a year and everyone tells me that I should be over my husband's death. I hold back my tears, but I still want to cry. I feel guilty that I still miss him.

- ◆ My husband comes home from work and I don't have dinner prepared and our home is chaotic because my son who is autistic is running wild while his older brother is watching TV instead of doing his homework. I feel guilty that I can't manage a quieter and more relaxed home environment for my husband.

- ◆ My husband was self-destructive. He smoked, drank, gambled and ignored our two boys. He died as a result of his lifestyle. I feel guilty that I am relieved by his death and that he will no longer set a bad example for my two young sons.

♦ I loved my husband and he died after a five-year struggle with heart disease. He was weak and a shell of what he was. He didn't want to live like this. After his third surgery, he died from infection. I felt guilty that during that time I admitted to my sister that I was tired of his illness. I feel like I willed him to die. Perhaps, I could have done more or pursued a different treatment.

♦ I feel guilty about switching to another doctor. I don't know how to ask for my medical records and my test results.

♦ I have had so many failed relationships; I will never find love.

Over the years I have encountered many women who feel responsible for their pain or their illness; somehow they should have seen it coming and prevented it. However, there is a clear distinction between feeling guilty and assuming responsibility for an illness. When we assume responsibility, we make every effort to heal the mind and the body. We partner our healing with the treatment. We don't fight the treatment or see it as poison. Instead we view it to be curative and yield to it. When we feel guilty, we disrupt our body from functioning properly and rob our spirit of its vitality. We fight the treatment and with this added stress, we throw our body off balance and make it harder for the treatment to work.

For example, because of the spiritual component of disease, some people are overwhelmed with guilt because they are sick and unable to cure their illness or that of a loved one's with their optimism or faith. They reason that their illness must be a Divine punishment because of a fundamental failure in their flawed spirituality. They conclude that they are simply not good enough or not happy enough and somehow deserve it. So, they beat themselves up over and over, ironically, impeding their own path to healing. They downplay the important roles of aging, genetics, environment and exposure to unknown toxins.

Consider this: Indonesia was hit by a devastating tsunami. Does it make sense to feel guilty, or say, *why me* when a tsunami hits? Is there any point to judging a natural disaster? However, what we can do is to accept a natural disaster, help rebuild the lives of those affected by it, and learn from the tsunami to improve the communication system to be better prepared in the future.

Here's how to be a realistic optimist

- ◆ Let your problems take a back seat. When a stressful situation arises, you can still do what needs doing, and be *reasonably* happy. However, you might have to yell at your problem from time to time: **Shut up!**
- ◆ Focus your positive thoughts on the here and now; concentrate on living your fullest and most meaningful life. Don't dwell on past or future loss. We all come into this world *in the middle of the movie and leave in the middle.* If you are cutting carrots, just focus on that action not worrying about the kids, your sick parent, or where you have to go later. Focusing on this purely physical activity actually provides a much-needed break from all your worries!
- ◆ Cut down on the mini-stressors of your life to help you deal with the bigger issues. You might not be able to clear the big stressor in your life just yet, but you can eliminate the little ones in order to generate more energy to deal with the big stuff.
- ◆ Channel your energy and direct it where it is most needed; prioritize your most demanding tasks when your energy levels are highest.
- ◆ Strive to be more creative in everything that you do whether it is a meal, a job, a relationship or a walk. Put

some spark into all your activities. Don't be afraid to leave your comfort zone to take a new job, get treatment or move to a new area.

♦ Pray in community to make you feel better and to help you to tap into group energy.

♦ Keep your hopes basic with realistic expectations: Get more sleep, eat balanced meals, see friends, plan an outing with the family, or take a trip to a place you have always wanted to visit.

♦ Make it a point to use coping humor. You can lessen the severity of a problem by laughing at it. Entertain yourself with your own thoughts. Think up amusing things to say as though you were a comedy writer. Humor generates hormones that have a health-giving effect!

♦ Worry less about the metaphysical why of things and concentrate more on making yourself feel happier today. No matter how hard we think and rationalize, we might never understand the why, but we can be grateful for what we have.

♦ Be kind to others. Be a cheerful giver and don't look to get anything in return.

♦ If you have had many failed relationships, work on making yourself the best you, so that you can have a healthy relationship. Keep trying to meet more people and this will increase the possibility of meeting the love of your life.

♦ Ease up on your grip to try and control things. When you yield to the problem or condition and accept it, you will have more energy to heal and find a solution.

♦ Clean up your home, get rid of the clutter and create a space that is inviting to others. This will attract positive people into your life to support and sustain you. There is strength in a circle of friends.

Meditate your way to optimism

Whether you are at home, at work, or at school, and you need to generate good energy, try Sister Peggy's *Five P's of Meditation* and you are good to go:

- ◆ Focus on the **passage**. This could be a quote from the Bible or any inspirational work like the lyrics of a song or poem. Even a short sentence that brings you peace can begin a meditation.

- ◆ Sit in a **posture** that is comfortable and feels right to you. Consider sitting comfortably on a chair with your feet rooted to the ground or in a half Lotus position.

- ◆ Create your **place,** a corner of the room or a small place on your desk. Make your place conducive to meditation; for example, position a flower, figurine, candle, or picture to release the relaxation response.

- ◆ Feel the **presence** of the Divine. Become receptive to the Divine within and without—allow this expansive benevolent light to gain access to your heart.

- ◆ Return to the **passage** to regain your concentration if you get distracted by people's conversations, the doorbell, telephone, or traffic; remember that noise is part of life. Don't get angry or feel frustrated. Become aware of the sounds and continue your meditation.

Exercise your way to optimism

If you are movement oriented and find it difficult to sit still and contemplate, consider a *moving meditation exercise.* When you focus your attention on your exercise and away from your worries, you are meditating! When it comes to this type of meditation, many people tell me that they are too busy, too tired or just hate to exercise, even though it has been proven to be beneficial to one's emotional and physical well-being. The key to exercising and even more important—sticking with the pro-

gram—is to find an exercise that: you enjoy, fits into your schedule and can be performed in a suitable and available location.

There are different types of exercisers.

- ◆ Type Ones are those who go to the gym, workout for an
  hour and then go home. They view exercise as pragmatic,
  generating good health and a good mood. Type Ones take
  different classes or exercise with a trainer to ensure that
  they are structured and committed to a time and place.

- ◆ Type Twos are those healthy narcissists who exercise to
  look good. Basically, they try to lose weight along with
  inches to fit into tight, youthful clothes and defy the aging
  process. A healthy narcissist cares about appearance,
  grooming and popularity.

- ◆ Type Threes are those unhealthy narcissists who are
  obsessed with appearance and applause. Some exercise or
  strength-train to the point of pain and exhaustion; some
  even fall into a pattern of over-training. Ironically, people
  who over-train tend to become depressed and their
  immune systems are weakened in contrast to the benefits
  that exercise is supposed to generate. Sometimes they
  even get a stress fracture because they have overtaxed
  their bones, muscles and joints.

- ◆ Type Fours are those who have a more holistic approach
  to exercise and select workouts that they enjoy and not
  something to get over with as if it was a punishment. They
  love to take a brisk walk along the ocean or jog in a park,
  play tennis, do line dancing, row a boat or swim. They
  have fun and cross train by trying different activities.

It's important to identify your exercise goals and reevaluate
them periodically. Write down what kind of workouts you are
doing and how you feel during and after the workout. If the
regimen doesn't feel right, or has become too routine, change it.
If you feel exhausted and achy, you are less likely to continue
exercising, no matter how good you think that it will be for

your mind and body. If you decide to go to a gym or community center for your exercise, don't select one that is difficult to
get to. Don't set yourself up for failure.

However, if you are having fun, feel happy during the session and energized hours later, you will make the effort. Soon
exercise will become an important part of your day and your
body will not feel right when you don't stick to your regimen.
Remember there are a great many options: dancing, sports
leagues, qi-gong, t'ai chi, yoga, pilates, stretching, strength
training, interval training, aerobics, martial arts, boxing, jumping rope, trampoline, bicycling, walking, gardening and fusion
classes which combine the best of many classes like a smorgas-
bord. Exercise videos and magazines which delineate the latest
workouts are readily available. Surely, you can find something
that fits your time and taste. Movement has the power to make
you feel good, liberate suppressed energy and make you
actively calm.

When you exercise, you set aside a concrete time to excel.
Your blood is pumping and your heart is beating; your mind is
clear; in short, you are poetry in motion. You learn to stretch
your contracted self to grasp your dreams. You give shape and
depth to happiness. And you thought you were merely walking or doing shoulder presses!

Self-care Mantras

♦ Happiness needs a sustained and continuous effort.
♦ Recognize what is before your eyes; then what is hid-
  den will be revealed to you.
♦ Channel your energy and direct it where it is most
  needed.
♦ When you exercise, you set aside a concrete time to
  excel.
♦ Stretch to grasp your dreams.

Chapter 10

LEAVING THE HOUSE

When Nora left the house to *find* herself, slamming the door on her comfortable life with her affluent husband and her pretty children in Heinrik Ibsen's *Doll's House*, the Scandinavian audience rose to their feet applauding the dawn of the modern theatre. However, in early twentieth century America the play's ending had to be changed to appease the audience; Nora returned home to her gilded cage living happily ever after. Today women are freer to leave unhealthy situations. In this chapter we will look at what happens when married women untie their aprons and run out the front door and what happens when Sisters exchange their habits for a secular wardrobe. Whether one leaves the convent to marry and lead a traditional family life, or one leaves a traditional family to escape a destructive situation, there is a higher authority one has to answer to: one's mother—alive or dead.

Tell your mother

I recall Terry, a tall blonde firefighter recovering from mesothelial cancer, sharing her story during one of my wellness sessions as she cried her way through a box of tissues. After 9/11 her husband, also a firefighter, was emotionally overcome by post traumatic stress; he was particularly affected by fellow firefighters who died during the attack. He began to drink heavily and beat Terry when he was drunk. At this time Terry became sick with cancer and realized that stress and fear were impeding her healing process. She began to suffer from irritable bowel syndrome as well.

One day she rushed out of our session barely saying good bye. She jumped into her car and drove to a cemetery in the

Bronx. The following week she revealed what happened. "I threw myself on my mother's grave and cried and cried. I begged her to forgive me. As an Irish Catholic, I was raised to believe that I was married forever and here I am planning to divorce my husband. I needed to apologize to my mother and explain to her that the man I had married was killing me inch by inch. And yet I felt terribly guilty." She wiped away the tears as she spoke.

Terry is currently divorced and feeling stronger and healthier. She is at peace with her decision, but her painful journey demonstrates the difficulty of leaving anything—a job, a marriage or a religious community. How do you know when to stay or go? You have to consider what you need to be happy and at peace. Sometimes in order to be loved we become chameleons in our environment, transforming ourselves into what other people want and wearing a mask so often that we no longer remember who we really are or what we want for ourselves.

Many of us cannot tolerate criticism and are frightened to express our personal style or assert our needs. As a result in order to make our situations work, we create a fairytale to romanticize the real facts. We make excuses and try not to feel our true feelings, but rather to feel what we think we should feel. Some women stay in an abusive situation determined to prove that they can be good wives and turn things around.

No Prince Charming

As Margaret's husband began finding fault with her, his remarks grew more sarcastic. She lost thirty pounds after hearing him complain that she had let herself go after having two children. However, nothing changed except that he began to find more things to criticize. Margaret felt her self-confidence erode and began to believe that she could never succeed in the workplace or even at home. "I felt like I was confined to the house and his limited definition of who I was. I felt depressed and could not tap into my creativity; I stopped painting. I became quieter and quieter as he grew louder and more offensive. When I gave him the silent treatment, his late nights at work increased."

Margaret began to have nightmares. A tidal wave broke through her bedroom window and inundated her living room with all the furniture floating on top thrashing around in wild energy. She awakened gasping for air. In another dream her husband had turned her into a prostitute and complained, "What a meager amount you brought in tonight. You can't even do that right!" Clearly her unconscious mind was trying to tell her in a flood of emotions that her husband was trying to control her through abuse. If she chose to remain in this marriage, she was the equivalent of a prostitute who receives no love, no respect, only fear and criticism.

The daily stressors will seep through the cracks in any romanticized story we try to concoct about our lives. Physical ailments like chronic fatigue syndrome, backache, headaches, or a more serious illness will emerge as a signal that it is time to liberate ourselves from the fictional story and face the truth: we can exist independently and support ourselves. We can show our children that we can learn from our mistakes and move on. We can't always fit into the conventional life we and others originally envisioned for ourselves. Charting a new course can hold the potential for greater fulfillment and joy.

Our unhappiness thrives on escapism like the archetype of Prince Charming. We want to be rescued from a vague, uneasy sense of our own personal needs and loneliness. We look to someone else to spirit us away from ourselves. However, if we are waiting for the Prince on the white charger, we might have to wait forever or marry our own idealized, romanticized version. The problem with the fictitious hero is that we eventually discover that the person we married does not resemble the one in our imagination. We fall in love with a lie and sustain it because it is easier to believe the lie than to admit a mistake and change.

To begin our rescue and bring an end to the staleness and intimidation, we need to exit our *house;* in short the house our parents built for us, the fairy tale house we built for ourselves, a prison with iron bars. This is not only a physical escape, but an emotional breakthrough. Consider the saying: *every exit is an entry somewhere else.* When we exit a bad drama, we are free to enter and get a starring role in a better one. Each challenge met strengthens our resolve.

Untying the knot

Sometimes divorce proceedings are prolonged—time is subjective and unpleasant time seems to last forever. The purpose of this exit journey is to recover our center, to become independent and to restore the balance in our relationship with ourselves. An honest reflection on the energy drains in our lives will help reveal what negativities within ourselves contributed to the disintegration of the relationship. These energy drains could be due to the childhood baggage we carry with us or the debris brought into our spirit by toxic people or events.

The divorce process is stressful because our significant other does not disappear the moment we separate. As the father of our children, he could be hostile or rude to us when he visits or picks them up. Legally, he might still be living in the same house until the finances and division of property are settled. It is important for us to counteract any negative energy with positivism. This is the time to keep our balance for our sake and for the children's.

For example, when Faye's husband arrived for a Sunday morning visit with piping hot coffee and muffins for himself, hot chocolate and donuts for the children, Faye was hurt and angry. She wanted to throw the hot coffee at him. However, she did not want to make a scene in front of the children who were sensitive to the situation and asked, "Where is mommy's donut? We can share with mommy." Faye quickly interjected, "I'm on a new diet and want to eat oatmeal and strawberries for breakfast. Does anyone else want oatmeal? The important thing is that we eat together and it doesn't matter if we eat different things."

Faye excused herself and ran into the bathroom and let the water run. Then she screamed. She focused on her breath, closed her eyes and breathed deeply for five minutes concentrating only on her breath. She felt her pulse slow down. She washed her face, fixed her hair and put on some lipstick. She returned to the kitchen with a smile. She made herself some oatmeal and coffee. She was no longer upset as she remembered this was why she wanted a divorce in the first place. She sipped her coffee and listened to her children talk about their friends and teachers. He did not evoke one angry word from her.

A tale of two sisters

From several conversations I had with the Sisters I learned that sometimes a nun needs to leave the community to which she has been spiritually and emotionally connected. For that perspective I turned to Mary Dever Kelly, Sister Peggy's twin sister who was a Presentation nun for a decade. Mary chose this teaching order because she wanted to be a teacher more than anything. During that time Peggy became a Dominican Sister, a preaching order, because she wanted to be a theologian. Mary remembered: "We did not see each other for two years and that was a particularly difficult separation because we were twins. When we met again, we acknowledged each other quietly, seriously and proudly. It was very dramatic and I will always remember our greeting: "Hello, Sister." It took on a whole new context." Mary and Peggy both felt fulfilled and happy about their choices; then ten years later Mary chose to leave.

This is how Mary described it: "I dedicated ten years of my life to the church and wanted to embark on a different journey. I never looked back or visited my friends in the convent after I left. I felt that my true calling was to teach, but initially my passion for teaching got mixed up with becoming a sister because of my parochial school education. I never knew a teacher who wasn't a sister. I continued to teach in the same school—no longer as Sister Mary, but as Ms. Tully."

Socializing and dating was a whole new arena—talk about being green. When she went to the Barleycorn Pub in Manhattan to catch up with her girlfriends from her *former* life, a man tipped his glass her way and asked with a broad smile, "Jack Daniels?" Mary responded, "Hi Jack, I'm Mary Tully."

Early on Mary realized that she could not return to her parents' home when she left the convent. Time had stopped for her parents. They still treated her like the seventeen-year-old she was when she entered the convent, but they supported her decision both monetarily and emotionally. Mary's mother put it this way to anyone who asked how she could condone her daughter's leaving the convent: *Mary can do just as much good on the outside as she could on the inside.* However, Mary explained that she was lucky to have such accepting and loving parents; other women who left the order did not fare as well. Some parents believed that by withdrawing their support, their daughters would return to the convent.

Leaving the convent is very similar to a woman leaving her marriage. Mary had this to say about sisters who stay even when they are unhappy: "Remaining in the convent, angry and anxious is the equivalent of a woman remaining in her marriage for the sake of the children. Eventually the negative energy is perceived and the children sense the unhappiness which trickles down to them." Anger and resentment wreak havoc on the body. It is important not to suppress emotions or to force yourself to fit in a mold that no longer fits.

For Mary leaving the convent was a life-altering decision. She married two years later and gave birth to a son. Sister Peggy's decision to remain in the convent helped thousands of people through her counseling and teaching. It is clear to see from these sisters' lives that you have choices and the personal empowerment to free yourself to take a detour or stay committed to your path—perhaps by redefining it and clearing the obstacles. The only way you can go wrong is if you do not honor your true, heartfelt desires.

Sometimes you have to lose yourself to find yourself

Jean Kawka, a former Dominican Sister, after high school graduation worked for one year before entering the convent. She dated a nice young man and considered the possibility of marrying him. In the end the convent won. However, with fewer restrictions, abbreviated habits, and changes in community life after Vatican II, Jean began to question the relevance of what she was doing. "I still loved the community, but I didn't have the patience to wait and see how the new religious life would evolve, so I left before the pendulum could swing the other way."

Jean adapted quite well to life outside the convent, but it left a void in her spiritual life. As a former nun, she felt anonymous at church and relegated to being a bench Catholic. "For awhile I stopped going to Mass. I felt as though it was a strained relationship. I was searching for my new identity as well as guidance from God as to who would emerge. I guess you could say the person who emerged is a composite of Jean and Sister Sharon Anne, my religious name. Now I am very much involved with my parish where I was asked to run for parish council. My parish is small; the priests know everyone by name. I found the community I was looking for all along.

"I don't believe I would be the person I am today—my faith and my involvement at home and at the parish—without having had the experience of being a Dominican Sister. In fact, I still maintain a close relationship with the Dominicans. Two special days stand out as the happiest in my life: The day I gave birth to my daughter Michelle, and the day I entered the Dominican convent in Amityville."

Before a woman decides to leave home, no matter the grandeur of that home, she makes a spiritual assessment. *Something is wrong here. The energy is different.* It doesn't matter what the reason is, whether it is an internal longing for fulfillment or an external conflict—both sides have to be *dancing in the same direction* in order for a relationship to last. Sometimes we have to give ourselves permission to walk away. It takes courage to follow new dreams. The unknown is risky.

This does not imply that we should run away from problems or adversity. Rather we need to be mindful, pay attention and take an honest accounting of what is happening. Some women are dancers while others are content to sit and observe. We all have our different roles to play. However, all women need to be alert to what drains them of their positive energy and to learn what will restore their vitality or else they risk becoming depressed, fatigued and sick.

The point here is not to feel as though we have failed or that we are quitters. When we process our pain, we learn from it and grow. We become more human and compassionate; as a result, our hearts can be more open to others. Wrestling with our doubts and emotions will help us to feel part of a larger world instead of living a small, limited and closed life. In the middle of difficulty lies possibility. Working on ourselves will help us to become more loving, confident and positive. We will then attract the love we need and the love we deserve.

How to prepare to leave the cocoon

♦ Take classes to pursue the goals and dreams you have postponed

♦ Plan to support yourself and become independent

♦ Express your opinions without fear

♦ Trust your intuition and energy levels

♦ Find a support group—positive mirrors help you objectify your conflicts and doubts

♦ Manifest your destiny: visualize what you want to have in life

♦ Honor your internal spark by not allowing yourself to be abused or neglected

♦ Be kind to yourself! Become your best friend

♦ Give genuine compliments to the people you meet. You will feel better when good energy rebounds to you

In any relationship there must be a balance between giving and receiving. If you are doing all the giving or the receiving, you will inevitably tip over. Come back to your center. Work hard to change personal habits to enjoy where you are or to leave an energy-depleting situation.

Recover your balance with process-oriented workouts

Training the muscles and the mind during a life-changing event provides an outlet for frustrations as well as the armor for self-empowerment. Because change is a process, it is a good idea to find a workout that is process-oriented and individualized to help steady the emotional rollercoaster. These workouts will help you to control your emotions, so that they don't control you.

♦ Martial Arts—the student progresses in stages. Movements are painstakingly learned in a ritual dance flowing one from the other. Martial arts utilizes both kinetic, rapid movements and static contractions for centered energy. The student learns to see the self and the opponent as a complement. Because the opponent is not really an opponent in this confined atmosphere, but rather your sparring partner, you will learn a great deal about yourself: your fears, conflicts, your reactions to the world and your self-discipline. Sometimes you absorb the attack and sometimes you use your own power to overcome your partner. Most importantly, you will learn awareness and self-control. The forms will teach you order and how to flow.

◆ T'ai chi—these exercises are more passive and slower than martial arts. Its movements are definite and invoke inner calm. The ritual, highly ordered internal movements flow and emanate from within. The purpose is never to stop the chi's energy or to inhibit its flow. If your chi is damned up and ready to explode, t'ai chi will release the life energy and help it to flow from the inside out.

◆ Yoga—its postures, asanas, are referred to as moving meditations. They channel strength and endurance in both mind and body along with flexibility. The Warrior Postures are excellent for changing directions. In Warrior II you look over your right shoulder which symbolizes your future as you look away from your left shoulder which symbolizes your past.

The added benefit of martial arts, t'ai chi and yoga is that they are all non-competitive workouts that tap into group energy. One progresses in a class with other students according to individual ability with improvement measured by personal accomplishment. A woman going through a marital or career separation will do better in a non-competitive, core training workout program where she will learn to be patient with the process of self-development and recognize the harmony available in daily life. She will also learn to flow more freely in a new direction. *Tough times never last. Tough people do!*

Self-care Mantras

♦ When we exit a bad drama, we are free to enter and get a starring role in a better one.
♦ We have to give ourselves permission to walk away.
♦ In the middle of difficulty lies possibility.
♦ Become more loving and you will attract the love you deserve.
♦ Manifest your destiny: visualize what you want to have in life.
♦ Tough times never last. Tough people do!

Chapter 11

NOURISHING THE BODY: SOUL FOOD

Hundreds of thousands of diet books have been published all claiming to reveal the secret to weight loss. Still our country is suffering from an obesity epidemic. Research shows that the more unusual the diet, the more likely we are to pursue it: Carbohydrates from heaven, carbohydrates from hell, cabbage soup, zone portions, raw foods, grapefruit, one food a day, fat flush. . . . We might take drastic measures like staple our stomachs or indulge in wishful thinking or magic potions to suppress our appetites and melt away our fat while we eat. There is even a spiritual diet where we pray that we can eat all that we desire and still lose weight. Those of us who opt to go hungry by drastically cutting calories soon discover that deprivation never works; in fact, we put on weight. As soon as we adhere to a strict diet, our obsession with food increases. The very nature of dieting compels us to think about food all the time. Therefore the solution is to stop dieting because basically we are not creatures of deprivation. No diet program has been proven to work better than any other, no matter how much it costs. Food is something we bless and enjoy. Any food that is on a forbidden list will have the opposite effect. We crave it all the more.

For example, the archetypal image of the apple, the first forbidden food, proves this thesis. God told Adam and Eve that they could eat anything that they desired in Eden. What did they crave? The only forbidden fruit—which didn't even come close to being on the same level as chocolate! Similarly, tell a child that he or she can eat any food found in the kitchen pantry or refrigerator except. . . . Well, we can predict the results.

Food contains powerful memories

Food contains many complex associations for us. For example, when I bite into a crunchy fresh apple, tasting its tart sweetness, perhaps I recall a personal memory of how I felt when I ate an apple as a little girl in my mother's warm kitchen on a cold fall morning, or maybe I see it as an archetypal symbol of the Tree of Knowledge, encouraging me to break the rules—again. I might remember my aunt lovingly chanting, *an apple a day keeps the doctor away* (which has medical validity). I might recall bringing my teacher an apple and placing it on her desk, hoping for a good report card. All of these memories flood over me as I choose an apple, wash it and ask, "Do you want a bite?" And here I thought I was simply selecting an apple rich in anthocyanins, anti-oxidants and fiber to promote a healthy heart, prevent certain types of cancer and improve mental ability!

For most of us food evokes comfort and security. Women find low carbohydrate diets particularly difficult because carbohydrates are emotionally satisfying and they raise serotonin levels. Chocolate, sugar and fat are especially comforting when we feel unhappy, drained, unappreciated and pessimistic about our future. Imagine a caregiver cooped up all day and night with an Alzheimer's spouse or parent—her only tangible pleasure might be eating creamy mashed potatoes, meat with gravy, cake and ice-cream; she is eating to fill up an emotional void. Bowls and bowls of cabbage soup will not soothe that ache—temporarily—like an ice-cream sundae.

If we are over-eating or eating calorie-dense foods lacking significant nutritional content, then we have to do some soul searching to figure out what we are missing in our lives. Most diets do not help us interpret the *why* of unhealthy eating—the reasons past or present. It is necessary to explore the following questions to make lasting changes:

Who is the person you are feeding?

- ◆ An angry adult who feeds off her anger?
- ◆ A rebellious teenager who feels the world owes her?
- ◆ An inner child who does not feel nourished with love?

Eating properly means paying attention to what we are eating and why we are eating. We need to make good choices every time we eat. Because we eat or drink something throughout the day, we need to be aware that we are eating and not nibbling without realizing it. We have to understand where our eating impulse stems. If we are stressed, eating will make us feel better only for the short term. We will keep cycling until we face the source of the tension. We need to fill up on good energy as we release emotional blockages. Eating huge portions corresponds to our greediness about the need to accomplish, or adhering to busy schedules as we devour time. Our greed extends to comfort and security, having developed an insatiable hunger for love and validation throughout the years.

When we practice reinterpreting negatives into positives, even those that occurred in childhood, we will learn to let go of all our suppressed anger. Presto! We discover that we don't need all that food or the wrong foods. If we give ourselves unconditional love and the permission to fail, we will succeed. The problem is that we are too rigid, too hard on ourselves. We don't have to be *super caregivers* to our children, parents, or the emotionally needy.

Tossing and turning leads to raiding the fridge—the midnight raid.

The same stress which prompts us to feed our anger and disappointment keeps us awake at night as well! We cannot separate our daily worries from our nights. Our overeating and sleep deprivation are interrelated! According to research studies skimping on sleep makes us more vulnerable to obesity. Less than seven hours of sleep sets us up for weight gain as well as insulin sensitivity. Leptin is associated with appetite control and ghrelin has been identified as an appetite stimulant. During sleep deprivation leptin levels fall and ghrelin levels rise. This could explain why tired people are likely to raid the refrigerator at night when they might be better off turning in earlier or sleeping later in the morning.

Sylvia, a high-powered Wall Street executive eats sparingly throughout the day. She skips breakfast, always on the run to catch the train. Her lunch is a salad with two cups of hot water with lemon, but no bread. She drinks hot tea in the afternoon and in the evening has chicken or fish with vegetables and salad and no carbs, but lots of hot water with lemon. However, she has not lost any weight and sometimes she gains a few pounds. What is the mystery? She confesses that she is a binge eater in the middle of the night. She wakes up about 2 a.m. every night worrying about the funds she is managing and proceeds to eat candy bars or decimate chocolate cakes! Her low-calorie eating during the day serves an important purpose: to enable her conscience to allow her to eat in the middle of the night! She would fare better and be less inclined to binge if during the day she ate more balanced meals consisting of protein, complex carbohydrates and healthy fat. Eating enough nutrient-dense calories during the day would stop her from waking up hungry craving comfort food. Balanced eating would help her manage her stress levels as well.

When the impulse hits, distract yourself!

When we feel the impulse to eat foods that are inappropriate because they play havoc with our insulin levels or clog our arteries, we can distract ourselves with a positive activity. We can take a walk outside to redirect our attention to the sights and inhale the fragrances of the natural environment. We can put on our sneakers and exercise to the music that we enjoy. We can work on a hobby and lose track of time. After mere moments our endorphins will be elevated and we will feel happier as though we had a chocolate bar—even better—because we did something healthy and affirming for both mind and body. We are transforming ourselves into the best that we can be. In contrast, eating the candy bar attaches feelings of guilt and failure—creating a lack of balance in our energy. When we feel an inappropriate eating urge, just calling up a friend on the phone can be an energizing experience which dissipates that craving because we feel connected, instead of isolated and negative.

The worst thing to do when a craving strikes is to turn on the TV and watch the endless parade of food commercials. The passive stimulation of the TV will keep you seated and munching unconsciously, like popcorn in a movie theatre—the previews haven't finished and that large popcorn bag is almost empty. Aside from the noshing, sitting all the time slows down our metabolism. So, we are eating more and moving less which means burning fewer calories. We need to move in order to boost our sluggish metabolisms.

Don't perpetuate sugar lust

The healthiest and most enduring food plan (notice, I didn't say diet) involves eating everything in balanced portions for the *individual*. For the most part our needs are basic, yet foods affect all of us differently and might not be tolerated by everyone. Generally, carbohydrates are an excellent source of fuel and energy especially before and after exercising. However, we should avoid the white kind. Complex carbohydrates provide a healthier and more lasting source of energy—remember it this way, life is complex. Whole wheat bread, brown rice, whole wheat pasta, oatmeal and sweet potatoes are excellent examples of complex carbohydrates that keep us satisfied longer by maintaining more constant blood sugar levels. On the contrary, sugar and white processed or refined foods cause sugar levels to rise and fall, perpetuating the cycle of sugar lust. Also, sugar is considered an inflammatory agent for the skin and internal organs. The latest cell pathology implicates inflammation as a root cause for diseases like arthritis, cancer and Alzheimer's.

The end result is that when we eat white processed foods and sugar, the pounds pile up; our skin doesn't have a healthy glow; the immune system is disturbed for a few hours; we are more irritable; energy levels drop; we feel unhappy and don't know why.

Feast your eyes

Nowadays our meals have increased to gargantuan proportions; we have lost the ability to measure with our eyes what a normal meal should look like. We are less likely to overeat using a smaller plate. If we are still hungry after having eaten a complex carbohydrate, salad, vegetables and lean protein, then by all means we can eat more vegetables and fruits. We can begin a meal with a big tasty and creative salad to help fill up before the main course and at the same time cut down on extra fat and starch calories. Drinking water before and after the meal aids in digestion and helps us to feel full and therefore eat less. Current theory claims that water speeds up the metabolism. Eating foods that contain water like soup, cucumbers, tomatoes, grapefruit, kiwi or watermelon fill us up even more than a glass of water.

Dining at a beautifully set table, with pretty utensils, a bud vase with a flower and a candle helps us feast our eyes before we even raise a fork to our lips. Add some uplifting music in the background and we are creating a delightful sensory experience. This sends a message to the brain that we are worth it. Chewing more slowly, pausing and giving our attention to the meal instead of eating while watching TV will help us to be conscious of what we are tasting, enabling us to feel satisfied. The mind and body are unified in the experience of eating.

Becoming aware of what, how, why, when and where we are eating helps us to make wise choices.

Small steps, giant *losses*

When we decide to make changes in our diet to lose weight, it is advisable to start with small changes and see how we fare over a couple of weeks. Slowly introduce the next change. If we overwhelm ourselves by cutting portions drastically, eliminating all sugars and white processed foods, we set ourselves up for failure. If we have been eating huge portions, cut them down by twenty-five percent. See how that goes for a couple of weeks. Gradually taper down and substitute more fruits and vegetables for potatoes and meat on the plate. Should we eat something sinfully delicious and inappropriate, we don't have to dwell on it, but can move on to eat healthier at the next meal. We don't have to give up and say, "It's all or nothing; oh well, poor me, I can't do this right!"

Shelley enthusiastically starts a fad diet every New Year's day. Two years ago it was Atkins with plenty of meat, cheese and fat, but no carbohydrates. This year it was the more expensive Zone diet which delivered small portions of food including snacks to her home each day. A serving of meat, chicken or fish was as big as a deck of cards. Shelley lost about forty pounds on Atkins over the course of six months and then gained back fifty. She lost about twenty-five on the Zone diet over four months and then got bored with the limited menu and gained back thirty. I visited with Shelley a few months ago and noticed that she had lost weight; she seemed more fit and toned. Shelley explained, "My doctor read me the riot act—my health was in jeopardy. My cholesterol was way over 300 and I was considered pre-diabetic. He talked about heart attack and stroke. So, I just made up my mind to get into my own "healthy zone" diet and I joined a gym. I may not be svelte, but I feel fit and healthy and I have a boyfriend."

Traditionally, New Year's Resolutions are filled with good intentions about diet and fitness. However, for many they rarely last. Either we make too many drastic resolutions to keep or the minute we slip up, we feel all is lost. I prefer not to make any New Year's Resolutions, but instead to make *evolutions* all year long. I am involved in a process, of turning the baser elements of my personality into golden virtues. Oh, and I never wait for New Year's!

Follow the Yellow Brick Road to the Rainbow Diet

When I was a little girl, I loved to read fairy tales. During the course of my childhood these stories began to shape my consciousness and inspired me with the magic of possibilities. I devoured books and looked like I devoured a whole lot more— I was an obese child. Reading was wonderful as it transported me to a world of magical transformation where everything was possible; however, the downside was that I became sedentary and hungry for wish-fulfillment.

Growing up as a child of two holocaust survivors, I certainly did not lack food. My European parents believed in the Rubenesque body and that my physical and mental health depended on eating all the time. Not eating everything on my plate threw my mother into a state of mourning. An obedient and sensitive, only child I kept on eating when I was no longer hungry. I lost my natural shut-off mechanism. The result was an obese child who felt different from everyone else—didn't quite fit in. I was called by a variation of my last name, *Eisenfat*.

The summer before I entered high school my parents shipped me off to camp for the first time. It was the turning point of my overeating and sedentary lifestyle. That summer I re-parented myself—intuitively. I began to think independently and broke away from the beliefs that were handed down to me. Parents, no matter how loving, could be wrong. That fundamental step of re-parenting myself helped me to metamorphose from a hungry caterpillar into a butterfly ready to take flight to other interests.

The next step I took was to eliminate toxic foods, like sugar, candy, ice-cream, and cake. I ate fruits and vegetables instead. I liked colorful berries and they had an extra benefit—slowly eaten one at a time. Then a week later I tackled portion control. I didn't skip any meals; but I ate about a third less and cut out big snacks.

Camp meant physical activity: walking from the bunk to the lake to the dining hall to the bunk to the playing field to the dining hall to the bunk. Then there were swimming lessons, various sports and even nighttime activities. The pounds were just melting away. I realized that just as in fairy tales, I too possessed magical powers! I felt lighter, more attractive and sociable, and I did a lot less reading.

Reflecting on this experience, I realized that a specific fairy tale shaped my consciousness about food and increased my capacity for happiness. My successful weight loss regimen was a combination of mind, body and spirit during a time when those three words were not fashionable. I followed a rainbow diet born from the *Wizard of Oz*, one of my favorite stories and movies.

Somewhere over the rainbow

Today I teach the rainbow food plan in my stress-management and wellness workshops. The Sisters love the simple, colorful concept and have fun decorating their plates with fruits and vegetables of many colors and sharing them with each other in the dining hall. There are many wizards out there selling quick diet fixes, magical elixirs and some of them are deadly. Each one of us has to embark on our personal yellow brick road to discover the three essential components of personality: courage, heart and intellect—the Lion, the Tin Man and the Scarecrow. Notice that Dorothy does a lot of walking on her journey and that's one of the best ways to fit in exercise and keep in shape. All you have to do is put on a good pair of shoes and walk out the door. According to trainer Frank Mikulka, "Exercise speeds up the metabolism. Exercise helps us to flow with life, to ease on down the road."

On the journey, we encounter both good witches and bad witches. These are animations of our personal attitudes. The good witch symbolizes our positive self-talk which is magically motivating and empowering. The bad witch symbolizes our negative self-talk which tells us we can't do anything right and that we will never succeed. During the course of our journey each one of us has to distinguish between these two voices in order to direct our attention to the chosen path.

The meaning behind the *Wizard of Oz* boils down to the power of perception. At the end of Dorothy's long journey, she realizes, "There is no place like home." We begin and conclude our search with our home—the body and the spirit. Each one of us needs to make peace with the self. *Home means being at home with yourself, comfortable enough to stand up for your natural, true self*—the way you act around others when you are secure and safe in your own home.

The premise of the rainbow diet is: "You've got to have some rain to see the rainbow." Adversity is a part of life; what we do with the pain, how we weather the storm, helps our inner light to emerge. Believing in the covenant of the rainbow restores our positive energy and capacity for happiness. When we eliminate negative distractions—stress, we will also eliminate what sabotages our healthy eating.

After we have made peace with ourselves and recognize the illusions in our lives, we are ready to notice the rainbow and experience it with our senses. Eating a rainbow array of fruits and vegetables—all the colors of the rainbow—we are sure to ingest the healthy phyto-chemicals, vitamins and nutrients to meet our daily requirements. Many of us go to the supermarket to shop for lycopenes, luteins, anthocyanins, anti-oxidants, cruciferous vegetables, etc. as recommended in the wide array of nutrition books. The rainbow guide is a quick, natural and easy way to eat healthy by choosing different colors: tomatoes, carrots, apples, broccoli, cauliflower, purple cabbage, spinach, kale, beets and sweet potatoes—no orange cheez doodles here. By filling our bellies with colorful fruits and vegetables, we can rest assured that we are getting more vitamin and mineral absorption than vitamin pills provide. Fish, chicken, meat or cheese don't dominate our plate, occupying a starring role, rather they might serve as a supporting cast.

Tips to remember about the rainbow diet:

♦ Get to the root cause of your personal stress. Re-interpret your perceptions to transform negatives into positives. Writing helps you to dig deep. If you have people to blame, write a letter blaming all of them. Now take out their names and substitute your own in their place. This becomes a different letter because you assume responsibility and no longer perceive yourself as a victim.

♦ Memorize an affirmation that has special meaning to you. When you memorize it, you can take it with you wherever you go—easily available in times of crisis. In fact, put an affirmation on your screensaver and tape a few inside and outside of your refrigerator. Choose from the many self-care mantras in this book or write your own.

♦ Get rid of negative self-talk. Instead, say, *I am filled with possibilities.*

♦ Re-parent yourself. You don't have to accept everything you were taught or handed down as sacred and untouchable. You are no longer a dependent child. Discover what works for you.

♦ Date your diet as though you were dating a boyfriend. Explore and get to know different diet plans and books. See what food combination works for you.

- Think of your meal like a decorator with an eye for color.
- Follow the yellow brick road—don't drive; instead walk, skip, jog or dance.

Follow this easy rainbow food plan to fresh air, warm light and a true awakening. Turn stress into a creative trigger to help you live your authentic life. Rediscover the truth about your core through your own personal journey. Please, don't wait for a house to fall on you!

Recommended foods

Here are some healthy foods to help you lose weight by filling you up and speeding up your metabolism when you eat them in proper portions. Aim for eating about six small meals a day to keep you fueled and efficient in body and mind. Remember that means small meals not full ones. A good guideline is to avoid eating foods whose labels list ingredients that are difficult to pronounce, for example, azodicarbonamide and arboxymethylcellulose. Some foods advertised as *healthy* contain a great deal of chemicals, hidden trans-fats and sugars. Keep in mind that asceticism and deprivation slow down the metabolism. You might be surprised by what is on this list.

- Peanut butter or almond butter (natural, no sugar) on whole wheat bread with a smear of all fruit jelly consists of protein, complex carbohydrate and fat. It is a balanced comfort food, reminiscent of childhood, filling and nutritious.
- Apples have plenty of fiber and fight cancer. Eating an apple before a meal will keep you from overeating.
- Nuts—almonds, walnuts, cashews, peanuts, etc.—provide healthy fat and protein and promote weight loss by satisfying you and speeding up your metabolism. Walnuts contain high concentrations of omega 3's, a wonderful alternative if you don't like fish!

◆ Moderate intake of (unsaturated) fat has been shown to be healthier than a low-fat diet for maintaining the good cholesterol in the body as well as helpful in controlling insulin levels by slowing down sugar absorption.

◆ Fatty fish like salmon, tuna, herring, mackerel and sardines, etc. contain omega 3's which are heart and brain smart. Your grandmother was right when she said *fish was brain food*. Note: that head and heart need the same diet to be healthy. Flaxseed oil falls into this category as well. Don't eat whole flaxseeds as they will be eliminated by your digestive system. Use crushed flaxseeds on cereals and salads or use flaxseed oil as a dressing.

◆ Whole grain cereal (not sugary ones) and fruit are heart smart and help you to begin your day right. Cereals are fortified with vitamins and minerals and have plenty of fiber; add some nonfat milk and you are good to go. Skipping breakfast slows down the metabolism and tends to promote weight gain. Your body needs fuel after a whole night of not eating and sleeping to begin the new day. Even if you are not hungry for breakfast, your body will adjust once you start eating it regularly and you will begin to feel hungry for breakfast.

◆ Studies have shown that dietary fiber including foods such as apples, barley, beans and other legumes, fruits and vegetables, oatmeal, oat bran and brown rice—clearly lower blood cholesterol. In addition, they promote regularity eliminating toxins from the body rather than allowing them to sit in the colon. In recent studies fiber has been shown to help control heartburn.

◆ Dairy products like low-fat yogurt, low-fat cheese, farmer cheese and nonfat milk, are rich in calcium which speeds up the metabolism and prevents weight gain around the abdomen. Enriched with vitamin D, dairy products help prevent breast, colon and prostate cancers. Also, these dairy products are important for preventing and treating osteopenia and osteoporosis. For those who suffer from gout dairy products lessen its severity and prevent a future attack.

♦ Eat cruciferous vegetables daily to boost your immune system against cancer. These include: broccoli, cauliflower, Brussels sprouts and cabbage. Broccoli sprouts are especially potent anti-cancer foods.

♦ Choose orange-hued sweet potatoes over regular potatoes which have more sugar. Sweet potatoes take top honors among vegetables. They fight free radicals to help prevent cancers and ward off illnesses associated with aging. They are high in vitamins A and C, potassium and fiber, but low in sodium. Vitamin A improves low light vision and keeps tissues healthy in the mouth, stomach, respiratory and intestinal tract. Vitamin C strengthens the immune system along with gums and connective tissues. And sweet potatoes don't have to be mixed with marshmallows or butter because they taste delicious just plain! One sweet potato is only 120 calories and it is a complex carbohydrate, so it won't spike your insulin levels the way regular potatoes do.

♦ By all means drink juice and get the juice machine going to experiment with fruits and vegetables. Popular fruits and vegetables to make your own tasty blends are: carrots, oranges, mangoes, melon, celery, apples, kiwis and cucumbers. When it comes to fruit juice, be aware that it is less caloric to eat the whole fruit which has water and pulp! The same applies to dried fruits which have a higher sugar content than whole fruit. Take care as too much fruit juice may cause diarrhea.

♦ For an alkalizing drink rich in enzymes, that is nutrient dense and won't throw off blood sugar, try drinking green vegetable juices like: cabbage, spinach, parsley, kale and watercress. If the taste is too strong, nutritionists suggest adding lemon, or some carrots and beets to sweeten it up. Studies have shown that dark, leafy green vegetables aid in calcium absorption. Kale helps to prevent age-related macular degeneration.

♦ Try to eat more raw foods—whatever your digestion can tolerate. Cooking destroys a good deal of the enzymes and nutrients. Certain foods don't need any imagination to eat in their natural state like fruits and vegetables. Other foods like meat and fish do. Remember that when you choose to eat raw meat or fish, make sure that you know the supplier and that it has not been contaminated by parasites or germs and that it has been raised organically. The safest raw foods are fruits and vegetables. Jack LaLanne is almost ninety and he is a proponent of eating five servings of raw fruits and vegetables daily. He juices a lot as well.

♦ Artichokes are low in calories, filling and take a long time to eat! They are a good source of Vitamin C, folic acid, magnesium and fiber and they are just 25 calories each.

♦ Drink about eight cups of water per day even in winter as a heated room is drying. Drink more if you are active during the hot summer. Water increases energy levels, speeds up the metabolism, flushes out toxins, hydrates tissues and helps fiber do its job. If you hate drinking water, add cut up strawberries or peaches to a pitcher of water and refrigerate. You will feel like you are drinking deliciously expensive spa water.

♦ Avoid sugary sodas. They really pack on the calories and have no nutritional value.

♦ Drink your coffee—in fact, the more, the better . . . In a recent study coffee intake was shown to lower the risk of liver cancer, Parkinson's and type 2 diabetes, and that was independent of a person's age, obesity, and other lifestyle factors that typically increase risk. Also, coffee contains many other ingredients that can prevent these illnesses, particularly type 2 diabetes—such as potassium, niacin, and magnesium, as well as antioxidants. Another benefit is that caffeine stimulates the burning of calories and may speed up metabolism by triggering muscles to burn fat and sugar more efficiently, prompting the breakdown of fat in other tissue as well. However, if you have high blood pressure or gastro-esophageal reflux—beware! *Personally, I'm going to hurry up and drink more coffee before the doctors change their minds.*

♦ If you don't like coffee, or seek a relaxing and healthy change of pace, try green tea. Green tea has tumor-fighting properties.

♦ Go ahead live a little and eat some delectable, dark chocolate. All chocolates are not created equal. Don't confuse dark chocolate with milk chocolate which has more fat as milk counteracts the benefits of dark chocolate which is rich in antioxidants and raises serotonin levels to lift your mood. To eat an appropriate amount of chocolate prepare a cup of hot chocolate or set aside a small portion of bittersweet chocolate for dessert. Don't sit next to the whole box—which requires superhuman self-control. The latest research shows that an ingredient in chocolate provides sweet relief from constant coughing, better than codeine. Also, chocolate does not make you drowsy, so it won't affect your driving or operating machinery. So if you have a cough, don't take a tablespoon of cough medicine, instead make yourself a cup of hot dark chocolate.

♦ Cinnamon is being hailed as a wonder spice: cinnamon can improve glucose metabolism and the overall condition of individuals with diabetes—improving cholesterol metabolism, removing artery-damaging free radicals from the blood, and improving the function of small blood vessels. You can use cinnamon sticks or sprinkle liberally with ground cinnamon to reap the benefits.

♦ While you are in the spice aisle of your supermarket, check out turmeric or curry which fights cancer, prevents Alzheimer's and eases the pain and swelling of arthritis and postoperative recovery. Use occasionally instead of salt and pepper in your cooking.

♦ Adding mushrooms to your diet is a wonderful idea. They are rich in selenium, a powerful antioxidant that is thought to help prevent prostate cancer. In addition, selenium is important for both a properly working immune system and thyroid. Mushrooms contain copper which works with iron to keep red blood cells healthy and they have B vitamins for stress management and mental acuity—all you need to eat is five medium-sized mushrooms to reap the benefits. Mushrooms are fancy additions to salads. Put them on top of baby spinach leaves and cherry tomatoes. Or shave some parmesan cheese on field greens and top with mushrooms, a little olive oil, black pepper and crusty bread and you're all set. Mushrooms sauté deliciously with onions and peppers. Sauté an extra amount to store in the fridge, so that you can spoon them into your sandwiches. Mushrooms are low in calories, high in vitamins and minerals—quite tasty. Cooking with them makes you seem like a gourmet. *Well, it works for me.*

♦ Certain foods facilitate sleep while other foods will keep you awake at night. Foods that are *sleep-inducing* contain tryptophan. Eat these close to bedtime: yogurt, turkey, bananas, figs, dates, tuna and whole grain crackers and warm milk *(your mother and grandmother were right)*. Other foods *will keep you up* as they contain tyramine, a brain stimulant—avoid these a few hours before bedtime: bacon, ham, cheese, sugar, spinach, eggplant, tomatoes, chocolate and coffee.

♦ Cranberries have been proven to keep the urinary tract healthy by preventing harmful bacteria from attaching to the urinary tract wall. And in this age of antibiotic resistant bacteria that's no small feat! You can reap the benefits by drinking a cranberry fruit cocktail daily, eating fresh or dried cranberries or even eating canned cranberry sauce. The next time you make yourself a smoothie throw in some cranberries. In your cup of hot tea use cranberry juice instead of water. To make a healthy topping chop one package of fresh cranberries, dice one orange and $^3/_4$ cup toasted nuts and put them into a food processor. Sweeten to taste and use with turkey or as a topping for pancakes or French toast.

♦ All berries are low in calories, high in vitamin C and take a long time to eat—one at a time. Their rich colors make them a varied group of phytochemicals and nutrients. Blueberries boost memory and keep the urinary tract healthy just like cranberries. Blueberries contain a compound that reduces cholesterol and unlike drugs, there are no side effects. Here is a serving suggestion to make a beautiful dessert. Layer pitted cherries, blueberries, strawberries, blackberries, and raspberries with low-fat lemon or vanilla yogurt in a sundae glass. Top it all off with a stemmed cherry. While on the subject of cherries, both the sweet and tart ones are being studied in diabetes prevention and management.

Add more fruits, vegetables and fiber to your diet

♦ For breakfast top your oatmeal or fiber-rich cereal with ground flaxseeds, almonds and berries.

♦ Layer the protein in your multi-grain sandwiches with tomatoes, spinach, mushrooms and peppers.

♦ Snack on: low-fat yogurt with fresh berries, a slice of low-fat cheese and a handful of almonds, cashews or walnuts.

Keep some dried fruit and nuts in your desk at work for when you get hungry.

Spice up your life for good health

♦ Garlic can be used as an antibiotic especially if you have a vulnerable stomach when traveling abroad. You need only to eat one or two cloves of garlic before a meal, or chopped raw garlic sprinkled over your food.

♦ Ginger improves digestion and makes a great tea to relieve congestion due to coughs. It also helps control nausea. Cut off a piece of ginger root and boil it. Adding honey is optional.

♦ Liberally sprinkle turmeric and curry on poultry, fish and vegetables to act as an anti-inflammatory and help prevent cancer and Alzheimer's.

♦ A handful of cilantro in your cooking detoxifies heavy metals and carries them out of the body.

♦ A daily teaspoon of cinnamon sprinkled on cereal, French toast or stirred in your tea helps prevent type 2 diabetes.

A little red wine and sherry are heart smart. I drink to your good health!

How to maintain your weight during the holidays

One of the biggest concerns hanging like a heavy cloud over the holiday season from Thanksgiving to New Year's is the 3,500 calorie meal. Many of us are worried about gaining weight and undoing all the hard work leading up to our dietary success. We fear that the meals, the parties and the office snacks will unleash a host of dietary demons as we revert to our old eating habits.

Who can resist that family gathering, with all the dishes slathered in butter, oil, and mega carbs with no one leaving the table for hours? Furthermore, many of us skip breakfast in anticipation of the big meal and that's a major no-no.

Let's look at some facts. According to nutritionists the more people at a table, the more each person eats—up to 76 percent more calories per person when there are seven or more at the table. To make matters worse, portions eaten with others are 44 percent larger and contain more calories than portions eaten alone. The larger the group and the better we know each other, the more we eat. Forewarned is forearmed!

So don't gobble, gobble; instead nibble, nibble. Here are some tips for guilt-free and healthy dinner parties:

♦ Eat a high protein and high fiber breakfast.

♦ Never arrive starving!

♦ Exercise the morning of the food fest. Make it a new ritual.

♦ Take a walk after the big family meal.

♦ Wear tight clothes. If you are eating too much, you will feel uncomfortable and be reminded to stop eating. Don't unbuckle your belt.

♦ Sit next to someone who eats healthy and is weight conscious.

♦ Eat smaller portions—a tasting menu.

♦ Remember that a serving from your hostess is not a portion. A serving could generously consist of a few portions. Know what a portion should look like and eat a small amount of that huge serving.

♦ Fill your plate with vegetables, and protein—no skin or fat on the meat. Chew slowly and enjoy each bite.

♦ No second helpings—except for salads (go easy on the dressing and skip the croutons) and steamed vegetables (sauces add up)!

♦ If you wish to have some alcohol, drink wine with your dinner and forgo high-calorie mixed drinks like eggnog.

♦ Drink water after the meal to fill you up.

♦ If you are preparing the meal: Serve dips made with non-fat yogurt surrounded by cut-up vegetables. Put more mushrooms, onions, celery, eggplant, etc. into the stuffing and less bread. In desserts that call for oil or butter, use unsweetened applesauce or pureed plums. Create a beautiful fruit plate, perhaps a pineapple boat. Serve sweet potatoes instead of mashed potatoes. And if you do serve mashed potatoes, put in some roasted garlic for flavor instead of butter. Prepare vegetables without oil or butter; instead sprinkle with dill and top with slivered almonds.

♦ Don't feel deprived. Savor a small dessert eating it very, very slowly.

The importance of the dinner ritual

At the same time that the family dinner hour is fading away, eating disorders like anorexia, bulimia, exercise addiction and the newest category, *mixed eating disorders,* are on the rise. Restoring regular family meals can help teenage girls and boys avoid dangerous eating disorders. It doesn't have to be a home-cooked meal either. Making family meals a priority, in spite of scheduling difficulties, consistently prevents eating disorders. Researchers suggest that parents keep conversation light and positive at the dinner table. Don't argue and above all, don't make food an issue.

Childhood is a mixture of memories. When we become adults, these memories turn into nostalgia which can be bitter or sweet depending on our experiences. What happens at the dinner table and family gatherings can potentially create emotionally charged experiences which will affect our lifetime eating habits. As parents, we must remember that today's experiences create tomorrow's nostalgia.

"Olfactory evoked recall" is a psychiatric term used to explain how memories are triggered by our sense of smell. Many of our own memories revolve around our interactions with our parents at the dinner table and therefore are linked with specific foods and aromas. If our past experiences were good: cheerful conversation, encouraging words and humor, we will have pleasant and healthy associations with food. However, if our dining experiences were negative: belittled, disciplined, silenced, bitter arguments, then we are likely to have problems with food. Family meals are a pretty good barometer of family interaction. The aromas emanating from the oven, the simmering pots on the burner along with the foods served on the table will forge unconscious behavioral associations with foods that will impact on eating habits and emotional well being.

Even if the family is loving and respectful, busy parents and rushed dinners do not create positive associations with food. It is worthwhile to consider scheduling family dinners and creating positive conversations to boost children's self-esteem. Children who contribute to meaningful adult conversation will do better at school and feel happier. Parents can use dinner time to establish rituals which reinforce their values. Treating a sickly grandparent with respect and humor at the dinner table sets a good example for the children. Remember: today's actions are tomorrow's memories. How do you wish to be remembered? What kind of adults will your children grow up to be?

An activity to unravel our complex relationship to food

It might be helpful to journal your emotional and physical reactions to certain aromas and foods. Emotional reactions could include: happy, relaxed, sad, nervous, angry, or rebellious; physical reactions: bloated, gassy, unappetizing, soothing, delicious, energizing, sluggish, or relaxed. Note the associations that come up for you. Observing the objective reality might help you to sort out your relationship to food, what you like to eat and don't like to eat as well as how much you eat of a particular food. Journaling your gut reactions might finally bring some clarity and most importantly, awareness of your eating habits, how they evolved and how they are triggered.

It's not just what you eat, but the order that you eat it

Every bite you eat, you make an important choice for yourself. The trick to staying on track is having healthy food available at all times. By scheduling a weekly shopping trip or ordering on the internet you eliminate food preparation problems. Having all the healthy ingredients on hand simplifies choices. Involving children in shopping and meal preparation gives them a feeling of pride in the food they helped to prepare. In addition, you are giving them lifelong skills and memories.

To keep your brain and your good mood well nourished, remember that the brain consumes 30% of daily calories. The brain needs at least 1200 calories a day for reaction time, concentration and memory. All meals should have protein, complex carbs and healthy fat. As I stated previously, small, frequent meals keep the brain well fueled with a steady supply of glucose, far better than three big meals a day.

According to Dr. Judith Wurtman of M.I.T. the order of the food you eat affects your mental state and has relevance to what you want to achieve. So if you want to be mentally sharp at work, pile on the protein first. If you need to unwind after a stressful day, fill up on healthy carbs first which will boost your serotonin levels.

The ultimate recipe for a healthy weight

Identify the situations and emotions that trigger your unhealthy eating.

- ♦ **Social** eating is associated with how we relate to other people. For example, overeating can result from nervousness, feeling inadequate, being encouraged, or wanting to fit in.

- **Emotional** eating can be triggered by boredom, stress, fatigue, tension, depression, anger, anxiety or loneliness.

- **Opportunistic** eating occurs because of the opportunity, a favorite restaurant, an advertisement for a particular food, the aromas from a bakery. Eating may also be associated with certain activities such as watching TV, going to the movies or a sporting event, etc.

- **Negative-thinking** eating to fill in the emptiness, a lack of self-esteem or feeling like a failure.

- **Physiological** eating is a response to the body's signals such as pain and hunger.

Distract yourself when the impulse to overeating strikes

- Visit or talk to a positive friend.
- Take a walk or go to the gym.
- Enjoy a bubble bath with candles and music.
- Using your 5 senses visualize yourself in a happy place.
- Do housework, wash the car, or garden.
- Dance to your favorite music.

Make small changes to your diet

- Don't cut out all the sugar, white processed foods, stimulants and big portions.
- Don't cut them out all at the same time.
- Do make a small change every week or two giving your body a chance to adapt.

Pat yourself on the back

Reward yourself with new clothes, a massage, a day at the spa, flowers, etc. Thank yourself and compliment yourself liberally for a job well done!

Remember this simple formula to maintain your desired weight: Calories in cannot exceed calories out!

The results of a number of research studies underline the importance of calorie reduction on weight loss and insulin sensitivity. *Excess calories in any form lead to weight gains and insulin resistance,* which increases the risk for type 2 diabetes. Therefore it has been shown that calorie reduction, not the amount or kind of carbs, has the greater effect on weight loss and increasing insulin sensitivity. From a practical point of view, a low-sugar, low-carb diet may offer a big advantage to dieters in terms of hunger management and diet maintenance. Complex carbs, proteins and fat are digested more slowly with less of an insulin response, which will delay hunger, making it easier to stick to the diet. Hungry people are not good dieters! Because carbohydrates raise our serotonin levels, which make us feel happier and stabilize our moods, we are more likely to stick to a diet that satisfies us emotionally. The good news is that calories do matter, so you can decide how you want to allocate your calories.

Now, throw away all the fancy, expensive and quirky diets!

Self-care Mantras

♦ Make good choices every time you eat.
♦ Dining at a beautifully set table sends the brain a message that we are worth it.
♦ Don't make New Year's Resolutions; instead make *evolutions* all year long.
♦ Exercise helps us to flow with life, to ease on down the road.
♦ Date your diet as though you were dating a boyfriend and get to know different diet plans and books.

Chapter 12

THE AEROBICS HIGH

Aerobics workouts are so much fun that we tend to get addicted to the natural high that is generated. Our bodies are moving; good energy is generated and our minds are carefree. We don't have to attend a special aerobics class to experience this surge of positive energy. Any physical activity that involves continuous rhythm is considered an aerobic activity. This would include dancing, step class, spinning, jogging, boxing, bicycling, gardening and house work—even cleaning and cooking. Pounding a chicken cutlet into submission is aerobic! Washing windows with alacrity is aerobic too. The key to achieving aerobic activity is performing a rhythmical, continuous contraction of muscles. This type of exercise increases the amount of oxygen available to the body—that's why it is called an *aerobic* activity.

Aerobics is also known as a cardiovascular workout as it increases the work of the heart and lungs. The CDC and the American College of Sports Medicine recommend 30 minutes a day of moderate to intense exercise. If you want to lose weight or improve your cardiovascular endurance, kick it up to 45 minutes or 60 minutes—6 days a week. For many of us the recommended time is just too much and rather than do a manageable amount, we choose to do nothing.

If you want to continue to workout, it's important to match your exercise regimen to your lifestyle, personality and fitness goals. Some of us prefer high-impact movement as though we were lifting off the ground while others enjoy low impact, more grounded movements which are kinder to the joints, particularly the knees. Some of us can easily schedule a 30-minute daily workout while others can barely squeeze in ten minutes three times a day. The great news: both are effective, healthy and have their own advantages. A 30-minute workout contributes to your overall endurance and gives you a greater aerobic benefit. However, three spurts of ten-minute workouts wake up both your body and mind throughout the day and provide a cumulative effect. Also, you develop a healthy mindset that exercise doesn't have to be an all-or-nothing proposition. It helps to define your fitness goals on paper and periodically review them to see if they still apply, or need to be amended to prevent burnout. Here are a few questions to ask yourself before you select an aerobic exercise.

♦ Where do you want to exercise?
  a) outdoors
  b) home
  c) gym
  d) the office
  e) all of these places

♦ What type of activities do you like?
  a) walking/hiking
  b) running
  c) sports leagues
  d) swimming
  e) dancing

♦ How much time can you set aside to exercise?
  a) 60 minutes daily
  b) 30 minutes daily
  c) 15 minutes daily
  d) only on weekends

♦ How intense do you want your workout to be?
  a) intense/working up a good sweat
  b) slow and controlled
  c) a mixture of the two

- What are your exercise goals?
  a) improved fitness
  b) improved appearance
  c) pain management
  d) disease prevention
- What kind of social environment do you prefer?
  a) alone
  b) with a friend or two
  c) a class
- How do you plan to maintain your exercise routine?
  a) take classes
  b) hire a personal trainer
  c) exercise with a friend
  d) schedule it on my daily planner

The benefits you reap from doing your cardio

Once you know how healthy aerobics is for you, both physically and mentally, you will make it a priority. The quantifiable rewards of an aerobics workout are that you will be able to work harder and become more active without feeling tired or overexerted. So, if your ship doesn't come in, you will be able to swim out to it! Running with a briefcase, suitcase, package or baby in hand to catch a bus will not leave you gasping for air. Your heart will work more efficiently at any given workload; your body will become more efficient in utilizing oxygen for fueling the activity, and your blood system will maintain a lower, healthier blood pressure, even at rest. Here is a list of just a few of the numerous health benefits:

- Reduced risk of heart disease and better heart function
- Blood pressure control
- Lower LDL blood cholesterol and triglyceride levels
- Reduced risk of stroke
- Reduced risk of osteopenia and osteoporosis

- ◆ Helps prevent and treat glaucoma
- ◆ Helps prevent and treat depression
- ◆ Helps prevent and treat type 2 diabetes
- ◆ Helps prevent and treat fibromyalgia
- ◆ Helps prevent and treat cancer
- ◆ Improves brain function
- ◆ Improves immune system
- ◆ Improves sleep
- ◆ Increases stamina
- ◆ Greater productivity at work
- ◆ Better control of hunger
- ◆ Less conversion of sugar to fat
- ◆ More muscle mass and a leaner body

A fascinating study of hikers in the Alps found that different types of exercise had varying effects on fats and sugars in the blood. Going uphill cleared fats from the blood faster while going downhill reduced blood sugar more. Hiking uphill or downhill lowered bad cholesterol. Hiking uphill is considered a concentric exercise, where muscles are shortened, as in a biceps curl or stair climbing. Going downhill is considered an eccentric exercise, such as when you stretch out a muscle, which happens when you step down. Researchers were surprised to find that hiking downhill removed blood sugars and improved glucose tolerance, while hiking uphill improved levels of fats called triglycerides. Now you can specifically target the exercise to treat your condition.

Aerobics can improve your performance at work

Those of us who regularly do moderate physical activity increase the *creative* quality of our work at home or on the job. Also, when we exercise vigorously, we are more pleased with our work and perceive ourselves as successful. And if we view ourselves as successful, then we inevitably fulfill our prophecies. Exercise sheds stress hormones and releases endorphins. Therefore when we are stressed at work or at home, we are able to alter perception and focus on the door that is open, rather than on the one that is closed. Cardio fitness transfers its skills to activities of daily living making us more efficient in completing our tasks. We have more positive energy and can literally whistle or sing while we work because of our increased lung capacity. Studies show that those of us who exercise during half of the lunch hour, for example, with a brisk walk, do not experience that late afternoon slump.

In contrast, sedentary obese workers had more difficulty getting along with their co-workers and complained more about their work; also they took more sick days. Their physically fit colleagues had greater endurance to complete their projects and were not as fatigued as their sedentary peers. To sum up: People who exercise moderately to vigorously perform better at work and have a better attitude. As a result many companies maintain a gym with trainers or offer a health club membership as a perk. If you work at home, follow the lead of companies by investing in exercise.

Okay, you are convinced and motivated to do aerobics, but how do you know if you are working your heart and lungs properly? I was never really good at math, but am still quite proficient when it comes to talking. Exercise physiologists recommend the talk test: when you do aerobics, periodically (every ten minutes) say a few sentences; in fact, they recommend reciting the Pledge of Allegiance. If it is too easy for you to say it, then you are working under capacity. If you are out of breath and have trouble reciting it, then you are overdoing the exercise and should take it down a notch. Find your level.

What will cardio do for you as opposed to lifting weights or stretching?

Cardio, weight training and stretching are necessary components of a balanced exercise program. (We will get to weight training in the next chapter.) It is important to understand what a specific exercise regimen realistically accomplishes in order to focus on what you are doing and evaluate how your fitness goals are being met. The specific benefit that you get from cardio is that it burns fat. If you want to burn the fat around the middle which increases the chance of having metabolic syndrome—proven to be a precursor to heart disease and diabetes—doing thousands of sit-ups a day will not help because there is no such thing as spot reducing. However, doing a cardio workout plus sit-ups will melt away the fat and sculpt your abdominals, particularly if you are eating healthy balanced meals.

The activity that burns the most fat is running. However, many of us are not runners, myself included, and in the long run our knees might not be able to keep pace with our hearts and minds. Therefore exercise physiologists advise us to choose an aerobic activity that we like because otherwise we will never keep it up. There are many alternatives and I recommend cross training to prevent burnout as well as constant wear and tear on the same joints.

It's not the exercise per se that determines the aerobic quality; rather it is how intensely you do it! For example, consider housework. If I am washing the floor or vacuuming, I can transform this drudgery into an aerobic activity depending on my speed and alacrity. If I put my whole body into washing the floor, cleaning windows, or vacuuming, then I am doing a cardiovascular workout. Try cleaning to the beat of fast music and really move your body! The same applies to gardening. Digging, cultivating the soil, weeding, pruning and fertilizing can become an excellent cardiovascular workout. Because gardeners love what they do, they lose track of time—to be envied by many dedicated gym members. I am so passionate about gardening that I have planted for hours in the rain! I can use this physical time to relax my mind from its worries.

Avoiding burnout

The next hurdle after you have committed to performing daily aerobic workouts is avoiding burnout which will quickly kill motivation. In order to stimulate the body and the mind you need variety. There are many options to create change: You can vary the workout, the intensity, the duration, the order, the location, the time of day and the music. If you workout in the morning and change to late afternoon, your perception and your drive will change too. If you take a brisk walk daily in the same park or track, then drive to another location and experience new sensations. Try mall walking during bad weather and use the stairs instead of the escalators. My daughter might balk at the thought of exercising, but demonstrates boundless energy when it comes to walking in the mall, trying on clothes and carrying packages.

Each of us needs to individualize our aerobics to enjoy the emotional benefits. For some people swimming in a pool for thirty minutes or an hour provides a lasting calming effect. The combination of the water and synchronized strokes or the varied moves of water aerobics creates a feeling of well being. For others it might be working up a sweat in an intense spinning class or step class that lasts for 45 minutes. The combination of the pulse of the techno music along with the desire to emulate the other participants both exhausts us and raises our spirits— it is what is known as a *good tired.*

A number of women in my gym, including a few grandmothers, love Frank's boxing class which requires boxing gloves and a focused mindset. They leave his hour-long class, sweating profusely and spent of their aggressions and tensions. One of Frank's *warrior women,* Fran, was going through an acrimonious divorce at the same time that her father was recuperating from emergency quadruple bypass surgery. Currently, she is moving forward with her life as she bobs and weaves the slings and arrows of outrageous fortune and counter punches each blow life deals her. Fran puts it this way: "If I can handle this boxing class, I can handle both my ex and my father!"

Exercise is effective in combating depression, anxiety and other mood disorders by redirecting our focus to the workout and to our breathing. Therefore the intensity and duration of the workout should correspond to the severity of the mood disorder. If we are mildly depressed, a half-hour moderate workout will suffice. However, if we suffer from more severe symptoms of depression and anxiety, then perhaps we should consider a longer and more intense session 5 to 6 days a week.

Even if you are a loner and self-disciplined, remember that group exercise has been proven to be more effective than individual exercise. In a class everyone is devoted to a similar goal; there is friendly support and social interaction. Exercising in a group may be exactly what you need to make fitness fun and consistent.

On the other hand, you might not enjoy aerobics classes if you are a rugged individualist and like to exercise by yourself. Classes might have cliques and women wearing tight, high-fashion outfits that undermine your personal body image because women tend to compare themselves to the most attractive person in the room. You might feel intimidated jogging on a treadmill in your sweats next to a consummate athlete. Bottom line: It's the fun and stimulation of your fitness routine that will keep you doing it. If you love aerobics, but hate the social scene, shop around for a few aerobics videos you can use in the privacy of your own home. You can practice the movements until you become more proficient. Should you choose to try the gym again, you will feel more confident this time. Sometimes the people in the "so-called cliques" are just as shy as you are about saying *hello* first.

If you have invested in a treadmill and are beginning to dread it, then put on an action movie or sports match like tennis while you are on the treadmill. The action movie or sports competition will get you excited and spur you on to exercise. You will lose track of time and continue to the finish line. I don't recommend watching the news or a cooking show while you are on the treadmill. Even comedies won't help you pick up the pace. Also, you can spice up your treadmill workout by changing the speed and incline every two or three minutes: walk briskly for three minutes; next raise the incline to walk uphill for two minutes; then lower the incline and sprint for a minute and repeat the cycle. Pump your arms, box in the air for an upper body workout while you walk. You can chart your progress. Remember to gradually increase your speed and the incline.

Tips for building aerobic endurance

- ◆ Maintain your workout for at least 15-30 minutes. Use the Pledge of Allegiance talk test to evaluate your intensity.

- ◆ If you are having trouble maintaining 30-minute workouts, try staggering three 10-minute shifts throughout the day.

- ◆ Exercise at least 3-4 times a week for lasting effects.

- ◆ Slowly increase your aerobic activities over a period of time to improve performance. Generally the more aerobic demands you make on your body, the stronger it will get. But be patient and increase levels gradually to avoid injury.

- ◆ Rest. The body needs time to recover and grow. Alternating more intense workout days with less intense workout days along with cross training can help the body rest and recover.

- ◆ Listen to your body: soreness, pain and tightness can help you decide what workout to do or not to do.

- ◆ Follow your heart: does an exercise make you happy or do you feel flat and spent? Don't do an exercise simply because it's in style. Set your own trend.

Warm up to your aerobic workout

A 5-minute warm-up will help you avoid injury and go the full distance of your workout. By slowly doing the easier movements of your activity, like walking if you are going to run, or leisurely doing the dance steps, you warm your muscles. They will be more flexible and prepped for a vigorous workout. A warm-up increases blood flow to the muscles and you will be less likely to experience the soreness and fatigue of lactic acid buildup.

Dress for success

Wear proper clothing for the location and temperature, allowing heat to escape or be contained. In cool weather layering works. In hot weather breathable fabrics are necessary. Wear shock absorbent, properly fitted sneakers and change them every six months even if they look good on the outside! Sneakers tend to fall apart first on the inside. Remember that your feet are your foundation and do the brunt of the work during aerobics.

Get fast music and change it regularly

Studies show that people who listen to fast music that they enjoy exercise longer before fatiguing. Even better, the upbeat music makes us feel as though the exercise is easier even when the intensity is the same. The American Medical Association has found that music together with exercise creates a synergistic effect which combats depression. Stimulate your senses with new music. Keep buying new, exciting CDs to help you to pick up the pace.

Experience a good tired, but no pain

Exercise can be challenging, but it should never be painful.

If you experience pain in your muscles or joints, stop. Give yourself a few days to recover, and ease back into it. For example, if you hurt your ankle, try RICE—Rest, Ice, Compression and Elevation. If it still hurts next time out, see your doctor and try an alternative exercise. Listen to your body. Don't override your pain with your mind.

Cool down and stretch

New research recommends stretching after physical activity rather than before. After an exercise session, your muscles are warm and stretching them will elongate them from their contracted state. You will have a long, tapered look. Basic yoga stretches have been shown to be particularly effective in reducing post-workout soreness.

Exercise reverses the clock

Aerobics will help you feel better and inspire you to take better care of yourself. There is a high correlation between not exercising and eating a great deal of fatty, sugary foods, watching more TV and driving to our destinations, even those that are just two blocks away. In addition, there is a proven link between psychological stress and biological aging. Caregivers of chronically sick children or parents are on average about a decade older than the rest of the population—down to the genetic level. I know of nothing more effective for reversing the clock than exercise. Shedding toxic stress efficiently and quickly, as well as strengthening the body—working out is definitely youth enhancing. Once you establish an exercise routine, your body and mind will crave it if you don't adhere to it. Exercise will add years to your life and bring more fun into your life. The race does not always go to the swiftest, but to those who keep on running. *Running for your life* takes on new meaning. Go the distance in good health.

Exceptional people share their workout miracles

Sol works out next to me in the gym on Tuesday mornings. He does the stationary bike and various weight machines. He is still driving at 95 and remarried ten years ago. He always greets people with a warm smile and interesting anecdotes. He checks if I am slacking off when our schedules don't coincide. "I haven't seen you lately. Have you been coming to the gym?"

Richard is 53 years old, HIV positive and has a malignant brain tumor which was partially removed and radiated. His oncologists gave him six months to live and advised him to get his affairs in order. However, Richard loves to run and maintains his regimen, some days running a little less or slowing the pace to a jog. Now, six years later, the doctors are astounded! He continues to run in the New York City Marathon. Officially, he is in what doctors refer to as an *indefinite* state of remission.

Michael, a national radio show host, was diagnosed with a virulent lung cancer. He was a smoker, but he also loved exercising and martial arts. After undergoing surgery and chemotherapy, he began to eat healthier and dragged his emaciated body on a stationary bike to wage a determined, physiological comeback. The doctors told him to write his will, but he just pedaled on that bike; suddenly he yielded it all to God. He made peace with dying while he was still determined to live. At that moment when he gave it up to God, he *felt* the cancer leave his body! "It literally oozed out of my body when I put it in God's hands." It has been over fifteen years and Michael is either in an extremely long remission—or cured, depending on medical semantics.

Marlene, a caregiver to a teenager with cerebral palsy, looks at least a decade younger than her 50 years. Although she is a devoted mother and takes her son to special, experimental treatments in Poland as well as cross country, she manages to find an hour a day to exercise. Her favorite workout is belly dancing, with her scarf tied around her hips she is good to go. She explains that belly dancing has strengthened her legs, abdomen and back. Also, it makes her laugh and bond with the other women in the class. "I can dance my feelings and release the sadness or I can be completely, joyously happy and not feel guilty about being so happy. Being fuller figured, rounded and having a bit of a belly are assets here. You know if belly dancing has survived over 5000 years, there must be something to it!"

Need any more proof?

Self-care Mantras

♦ Performing moderate physical activity will increase the creative quality of your work.
♦ Match your exercise regimen to your lifestyle, personality and fitness goals.
♦ When it comes to exercising, be an individual and set your own trend.
♦ Music together with exercise creates a synergistic effect to combat depression.
♦ Exercise will add years to your life and life to your years.

Chapter 13

THE CHANGING HABITS PROGRAM

Before You Begin This Exercise Program

♦ Consult your doctor. Know that you perform these exercises at your own risk.

♦ Fit in Fitness: schedule your workout sessions on a calendar visible to all family members.

♦ Maintain a balanced diet to fuel your muscles and enhance overall body health.

♦ Drink plenty of water to prevent dehydration and help flush out toxins.

♦ Maintain proper body alignment when executing an exercise; a mirror can help.

♦ Do not use momentum. Do each repetition slowly and carefully with a steady and controlled speed of movement.

♦ Hold abdominals in tightly to support the back and create core stability.

♦ Don't hold your breath. Breathe rhythmically, exhaling on exertion.

♦ Maintain focus by visualizing the working muscle.

♦ Stop if you feel any pain or dizziness. Distinguish pain from a *burn* that is felt in the last few repetitions of weight training.

♦ Make sure to stretch to lengthen the muscle after your workout to increase flexibility and prevent injury to muscles and connective tissue.

- Incorporate rest periods (a day or two) when strength training. Let muscles recover and repair. On rest days, known as *active rest*, take a walk, swim, or take a dance class.
- Create a balanced program alternating between weight training and cardio components.
- Keep advancing in your workouts and change them periodically to stimulate your body and promote development. The body adapts to continued routines.
- Have fun!

How long? How Often? Where? What Do I Need?

The exercise sequence of the *Changing Habits* program is designed to flow from one movement to the next: From large muscle groups to small ones. Also, the exercise order can be reversed and personalized. One session might begin with the chest working your way down the body and the next session might begin with squats working up to the chest. Allow 30 - 45 minutes for the exercises. Do the program 2 to 3 times a week.

However, if you only have a few minutes, then get fit fast! Take your workout to the max!

Do the following 3 exercises as shown in the program:

- Push-ups to work your upper body
- Abdominals to strengthen your core
- Squats to work your lower body

Or you can do

- One arm low rows to work your back
- Rear lunges for your lower body
- Wall marches for lower body strength and endurance

In this short span of time you are exercising several large major muscle groups and performing compound movements. Compound exercises also correspond more realistically to activities of daily living and will help you to function better with greater strength and balance. To speed things up you can do one set of each exercise as opposed to two sets. In this way you are cutting repetitions, not body parts because you are doing one exercise per body part. In strength training you always strive for body balance—no weak link. Although ten minutes is not a big investment in time, you will reap a lot of dividends! Less can be more.

The goal is progressive resistance. When the workout gets easier, you can change the

- ◆ Speed—slower is harder
- ◆ Sequence of the exercises
- ◆ Intensity—as soon as 12 repetitions (the number of times you lift a weight within a set of exercises) feel easy, then increase the weight and do 8 repetitions—building up to 12.

Change will stimulate your muscles to continue to grow stronger. You can pick up the pace by creating aerobic intervals. Instead of concluding with wall marches, begin with them and incorporate them for 1-2 minute intervals between the strength-training exercises.

Use the *Changing Habits* program to jumpstart your fitness level and your life. You don't need a gym or expensive equipment to take back your power. All you will need for your workout: a carpeted floor or a mat, a pair of dumbbells, a ball and/or medicine ball, empty plastic laundry detergent bottles, a sturdy chair and a couch. Turn on the phone machine to screen your phone calls and play your favorite upbeat music.

Please join Frank Mikulka, Sister Peggy Tully and me in the exercises demonstrated in the following pages and invest in your health and energy levels. We guarantee a few smiles among the grunts and groans.

Push-ups

You are working your chest muscles and triceps while emotionally learning to open your heart.

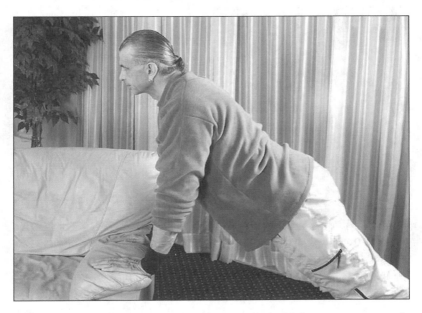

Do a set of push-ups off the arm of your couch. Make sure your couch rests firmly against the wall (at least on one side), so that it does not slide. Note the start position: Back is straight; abdominals are tight and hands are positioned directly under your shoulders with fingers facing forward. Extend your body full length with your weight on your toes.

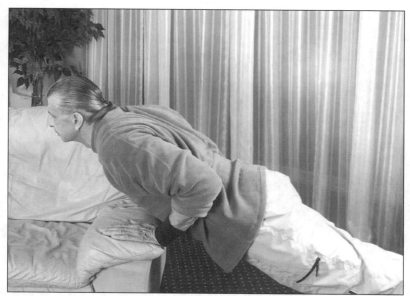

Lower your chest to the arm of the couch by bending your elbows (do not lock them out) which point back as your hands rest alongside your chest. Your eyes look straight ahead as you keep your neck in line with your spine; hold for 2 counts and then lift up again to the start position. Exhale on exertion. Remember to maintain a flat back and tight abdominals. Do a set of 5 repetitions. Don't rush. Work your way up to 2 sets of 10.

Floor Chest Press

We follow the push-up with a floor chest press to do some more upper body work—an area generally under-worked in women. This is known as a compound set because we are still working the same group of chest muscles we did in the push-up. Note: You also have the option to choose the order of the chest press or the push-up to vary the exercise. Changing your routine wakes up the body and triggers new muscle tissue growth. After this exercise, your heart will be more open to love and friendship.

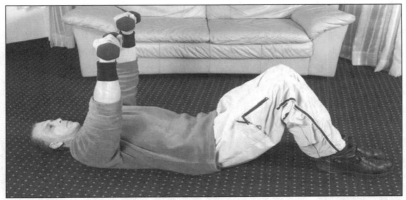

In the start position lie down on the floor with a dumbbell in each hand (weight determined by you, suggested starting weight 5 lbs; most advanced all the way up to 12 lbs or weight where you execute without breaking form) and knees bent; keep your wrists straight, neutral with hand and elbow in a straight line, throughout the move. Inhale as you extend both arms straight up from your shoulders and in line with your chest.

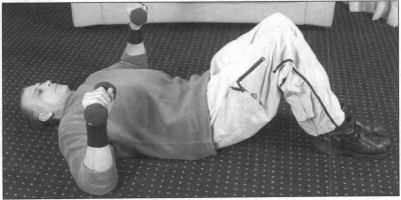

Next bend at the elbows as you lower. Stop when you feel contact with the floor. Exhale through the mouth, pursed lips, on exertion— the part of the movement requiring the most effort. Then return to start and extend your arms up towards the ceiling. Try to do a set of 5-8 repetitions. Work your way up to 2 sets of 10-12. When this feels easy, increase the weight of your dumbbells.

Abdominals

While we are still on the floor, let's work on our core by doing abdominals. Strong abdominals will protect your back and help you maintain good core balance. In fact, you can work your abdominals in every exercise you do. Make sure to pull them tightly into your back for core stability. The branches of a tree are as strong as its trunk.

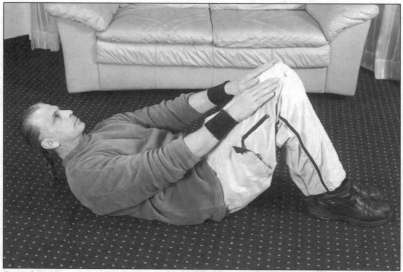

Lie down on the floor with your knees bent and arms at your sides. Contract your abdominals by pulling your navel in towards your spine, press your back down into the floor and then lift your shoulders off the floor: Think **contract, compress,** (flex spine) **and lift.** Remember to exhale on exertion. When you lift from the abdominals, paint your thighs with your hands. Eyes look up. You should be able to put an orange under your chin. Do quality repetitions. This is not a sit-up test. Do them slowly and controlled. Make each one count! Aim for 3 sets of 15.

One Arm Low Rows

What has a front has a back. So let's work our back muscles by doing one arm low rows with our easy-to-grip gallon laundry detergent containers.

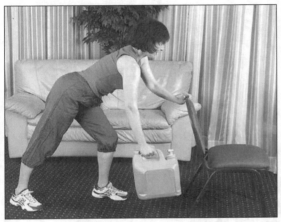

Fill the container with enough water to make it challenging, but comfortable to lift. Use a sturdy chair for support and bend your left knee. The right leg extends behind you. Contract your abdominals and make sure that your back is flat. Shoulders are back and the right arm is extended; wrist is straight, neutral with hand and elbow in a straight line. This is your start position.

Next, pull your arm, so that your elbow goes beyond your back. Feel the middle of your back contract as you hold this position for 2 counts. The arm movement simulates a sawing motion. Then return to start position. Do 8 repe-

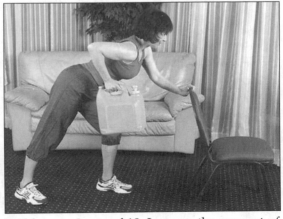

titions on each side. Build up to 3 sets of 10. Increase the amount of water in your container when the exercise feels easy.

Side Laterals

Shoulders bear a lot of responsibility; remember that it is not the load that you carry, but the way you carry your load.

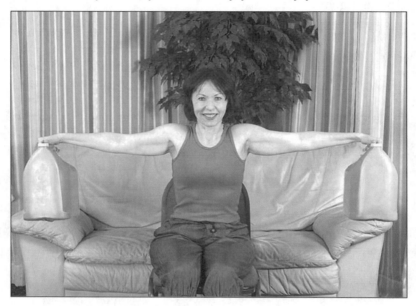

Instead of using 3-5 lb dumbbells, let's get creative. Try using empty laundry detergent bottles with handles as free weights. Fill them with the amount of water that feels comfortable for lifting. Sit on a chair or you can stand. With both arms down at your sides, lift to shoulder height, extending both arms, but do not hyperextend. Keep your wrists straight, neutral with hand and elbow in a straight line. Remember to breathe. Then lower to your sides. Do not swing the weights. Do a set of 8-10. Then hold for 10 seconds in an iron cross position to break momentum. Continue for two more repetitions. Advance to 3 sets of 10 repetitions. When that feels easy, increase dumbbell weight or add more water to make the detergent bottles heavier.

Shoulder Presses

To vary your shoulder work you can choose to do a shoulder press.

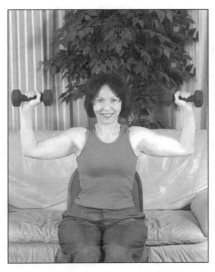

If you have dumbbells, then you can go the conventional route. You can do this exercise seated or standing. Pick up a pair of dumbbells (weight determined by you, suggested starting weight 3-5 lbs) and using an overhand grip, hold your wrists straight, neutral with hand and elbow in a straight line, perpendicular to your elbows. The dumbbells should be level with your ears. Hold your abdominals in tightly.

Push straight up from the elbows and don't hyperextend. Keep your elbow joint soft on the up-phase in order not to lock out the joint. Don't touch the dumbbells together at the top. Exhale on exertion. Then return to start position. Do a set of 10 shoulder presses, gradually advancing to 3 sets of 12. When this feels easy, increase your weight to what's comfortable. Don't rush; make sure to execute controlled movements.

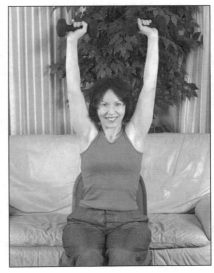

Biceps Curls

Another way to carry our load is to use the biceps muscles. We use our biceps to carry our children, groceries and aging parents—and now and then for shopping at the mall.

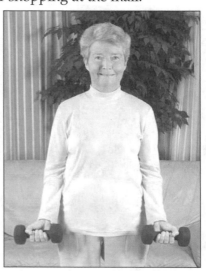

To start: Stand with feet firmly planted, hip distance apart, a slight bend in the knees. Relax your knee-joint. Keep your elbows stationary at your sides. Hold your dumbbells (weight determined by you, suggested 3-8 lbs) with palms facing forward. Abdominals are tight.

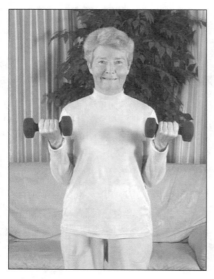

Now lift the weight up to your chest. Exhale on exertion. Do not use your wrist, but lift and lower from the biceps. Return to the start position which is a full extension. Do not use momentum or rock your body. Maintain core stability. To challenge yourself midway through the set, hold the biceps curl at chest level for 10 seconds and then complete your set. Do a set of 10 repetitions. Aim for 2 sets of 10. When this feels easier, increase the weight of your dumbbells.

Ball Biceps Curls

Tired of your dumbbells? Be inventive!

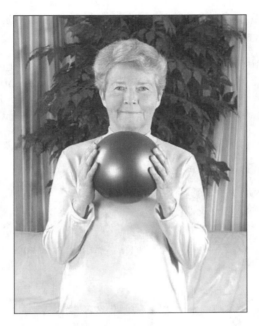

You can choose a weighted ball for your biceps curls—same instructions as for your free weights. Every change wakes up both your muscle and your mind and gives you some variety in your program. When this feels easy, get a heavier medicine ball.

Triceps Dips

Let's work the triceps muscles next, the opposing muscle group to the biceps, and the part of the arm for which women have the most trouble getting enough exercise. Also, it jiggles when we wave to our friends.

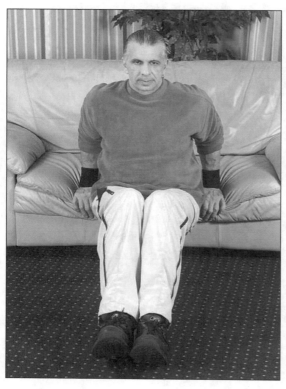

Use your own body weight for resistance. Holding on to a stable piece of furniture like a couch or a coffee table, place your hands directly outside your hips, palms facing down. Keep your buttocks close to the edge of the couch and bend your knees as you slowly lower your body to the floor as you bend your elbows behind you. Let your upper arms and forearms form a right angle. Pause at the bottom; exhale on exertion. Then slowly lift your body to where you began by straightening your arms. Do 10 repetitions per set. Aim for 2 sets. Note: the closer your legs are to your body, the easier the triceps dip. The farther away your legs, the more stress you place on the triceps muscle and this makes the dip harder to do. When this feels easy, simply move your legs farther out.

Double Ball Squeeze

As we make the transition from upper to lower body, here is an excellent move to incorporate both for total body fitness: chest, arms and inner thighs.

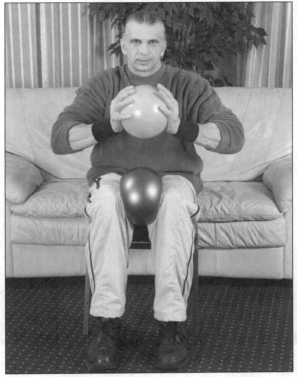

Sit on a sturdy chair and use two soft balls. Simultaneously squeeze one with arms bent, both palms pressing the ball at chest level to work the chest and biceps and squeeze the other ball between your thighs to work your inner thighs. Maintain core stability. Squeeze the balls with a pulsating rhythm. Exhale on exertion. Squeeze hard. Try to do 5 repetitions. Hold tightly on the last one for 5 seconds. Aim for 3 sets of 5 repetitions. When this feels easy, increase the repetitions and hold the last one for 10 seconds.

Squats

The squat is a multi-joint exercise for the lower body involving the hips, legs and buttocks. It increases balance and will build bone mass in the hips. Take it to the next level using your broom, body bar or barbell. Don't be a desperate housewife; transform yourself into warrior woman and sweep away the obstacles in your path.

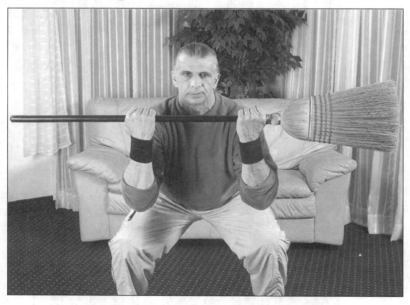

Make sure that your heels stay on the floor as you squat to sit on an imaginary chair. The lower you squat, the more you recruit your glutes. Hold your abdominals tightly and push off your heels. Holding the broom recruits your biceps muscles and keeps you in good alignment for your squat; you get two exercises for the price of one. Exhale on exertion. Rise to your full height; your arms hold the broom throughout the movement and then repeat. Try to do a set of 10 repetitions. Aim for 3 sets. Progression is: broom to weighted body bar to dumbbells or barbell.

Having-a-ball Squats

Here's a total body movement involving the squat. You are working just about everything! You will reap some cardio benefit here while you have a ball.

Place a ball on the floor in front of you and get into squat position, heels firmly planted. Bend, pick up and reach.

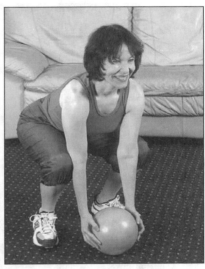

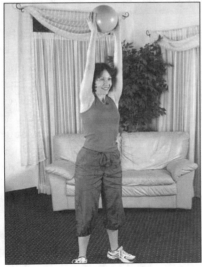

From a squat position pick up the ball from the floor, hold it in front of your chest (not shown). Pushing off your heels, stand up and lift your arms to place the ball high overhead on an imaginary shelf. Exhale on exertion. Do a set of 10. Aim for 2 sets of 12. When this feels easy, use a weighted medicine ball.

Reverse Lunges

Reverse lunges will strengthen your quadriceps muscles with less stress on the knee joint to help you walk forward to your next happiness.

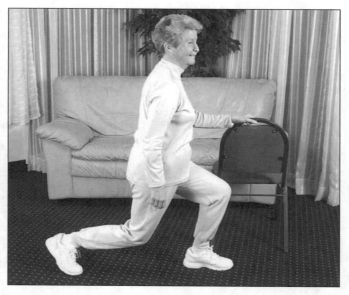

Stand up straight and tall with abdominals tight and both legs together (not shown). Hold on with one hand to a sturdy chair for balance. Take a slow and controlled step back with one leg, balancing yourself on the ball of your foot. Bend both knees as you lower your hips toward the floor. Make sure not to let the back knee touch the floor, or to let your front knee extend over your toes. Push off the leg that is behind you and your front heel; exhale on exertion. Return to start position with both legs together. Do 2 sets of 8-10 on each leg. When this feels easy, don't hold on to the chair. Progress to alternating lunges.

Lunge Torso Twist

As long as I have you in a lunging mood, and you are getting accustomed to doing lunges, get your ball and let's do a more advanced compound move, known as a lunge torso twist. This will strengthen your back muscles, abdominals, hips and legs for core stability and power.

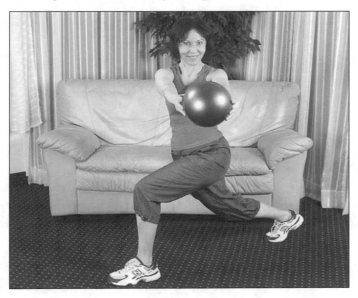

Get your ball and stand in a lunge position. Tighten your abdominals and hold the ball out in front of your chest. Twist in the direction of the foot that is firmly planted in front of you. Dig in to keep your balance. Keep your eye on the ball. Maintain lunge position and twist again to the same side. Do a set of 8. Then switch legs and repeat on the other side. Build up to 2 sets of 10 and when this feels easy, use a weighted medicine ball.

Leg Extensions

Let's strengthen the quadriceps and take the stress off the hip joint with seated leg extensions.

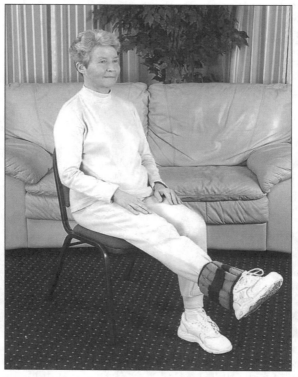

Sit on a sturdy chair and strap on an ankle weight of 2 lbs. Flex your foot and extend your leg out in front. Do not hyperextend your knee or lock it out—keep the knee soft. Tighten your thigh muscle. Remember to exhale on exertion. Bend your knee and lower your leg back down to the start position. Do a set of 10 on each leg. Aim for 2 sets. When this feels easy, increase the ankle weight to 3 then 5 lbs.

Leg Curl

We don't want to tip over, so after we strengthen our quadriceps, it is time to strengthen our hamstrings with a rear leg curl. Strong hamstrings also protect the knee.

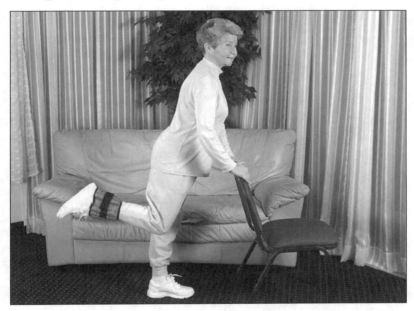

Since you are still wearing your ankle weight, hold on to a sturdy chair, feet planted about a foot behind the chair. Tighten your abdominals. Balance your weight on one leg as you bend at the knee and curl up the leg wearing the ankle weight to your buttocks to form a right angle. Tighten your hamstring as you curl up. Exhale on exertion. Then return to start position. Do a set of 10 repetitions and then switch legs. Aim for 2 sets. When this feels easy, increase the ankle weight 3-5lbs.

Side Leg Lifts

While I'm in the neighborhood, for the sake of balance, let's do some side leg lifts for the outer thighs and hips. Hint: When you are stuck waiting in an office with nothing to do, you can subtly do these against the wall.

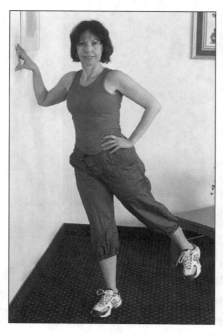

Stand next to the wall for support. Shift your body weight to the foot nearest the wall. Lift and extend your other leg to the side slightly behind you with your toes pointing down. Hold for 2 counts. Keep your abdominals tight and exhale on exertion. Then return to start position with both feet placed under your hips. Do a set of 10-12 and then switch sides. Aim for 3 sets per leg. Hint: Imagine a weight on your ankle while lifting to mind the muscle you are working. To take it to the next level you can wear your ankle weight.

Calf Raises

No leg workout is complete without getting the blood pumping into your calves. Calf raises will help you go the distance and you won't need to wear high heels to look good on your journey! You can subtly do them while you wait on line with your shopping cart in the supermarket.

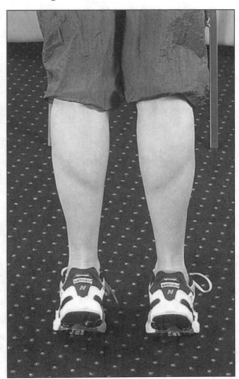

Hold on to the back of a sturdy chair, legs stretched behind you. Rise on the balls of your feet, lifting your heels off the floor. Concentrate on pushing off the big toe and ball of the foot. Keep your alignment through instep and ankle. Exhale on exertion. Hold for 2 counts and then lower your heels back to the floor. Do a set of 10-12. Aim for 3 sets of 12. When this feels easy, increase the repetitions.

Wall Marches

Don't be a wall flower! Conclude with a wall march. Imagine a marching band announcing the successful completion of your workout, ending on an aerobic high! Note: you can use wall marches as a cool down or warm-up; choose how you begin and how you end!

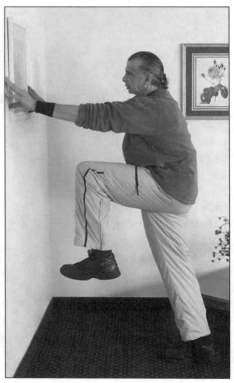

Stand with your feet shoulder width apart and position your hands the same distance lightly touching the wall for stability. Hold your abdominals tight. Then lift your leg high to your waist, forming a right angle. Exhale on exertion. Do alternate leg lifts and aim for 3 sets of 20 or more. When this feels easy, do wall marches between exercises.

OTHER BOOKS OF INTEREST

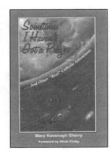

SOMETIMES I HAVEN'T GOT A PRAYER
... And Other "Real" Catholic Adventures
Mary Kavanagh Sherry

"... down-to-earth, even extremely funny, and filled with insights born of love and lighthearted determination to be a growing yet faithful believer committed to Catholicism."
—*Dominican Vision*

No. RP 174/04 ISBN 1-878718-79-7   **$8.95**

THE POWER OF ONE
Christian Living in the Third Millennium
Msgr. Jim Lisante

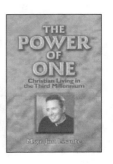

"Many of the stories could be used in counselling sessions, religious education classes, or Bible studies as explorations of love, compassion, anger, frustration and caring. The stories are short but have deep meaning." —**Crux of the News**

No. RP 180/04 ISBN 1-878718-84-3   **$9.95**

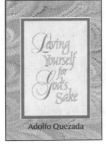

LOVING YOURSELF FOR GOD'S SAKE
Adolfo Quezada

This exquisite book of meditations gently directs the reader to see the gift of self in an entirely new and beautiful light. It presents a spirituality of self-love not based on narcissism, but as a response to the divine invitation to self-nurturing.

No. RP 720/04 ISBN 1-878718-35-5   **$5.95**

A PARTY OF ONE
Meditations for Those Who Live Alone
Joni Woelfel

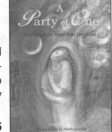

Using each day's brief reflection, probing question and pertinent quote by Adolfo Quezada, this book will comfort and empower those living alone to take ownership for their life, confident of being guided and upheld by God.

No. RP 744/04 ISBN 1-933066-01-6   **$5.95**

OTHER BOOKS OF INTEREST

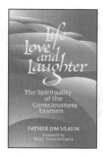

LIFE, LOVE AND LAUGHTER
The Spirituality of the Consciousness Examen
Father Jim Vlaun

"Within only a few pages, you know you're in the company of a truly good man, someone with a big heart whose feet are firmly on the ground . . . There is so much simple, shining wisdom in this book." **—William J,. O'Malley, S.J.**
No. RP 113/04 ISBN 1-878718-43-6 **$7.95**

HEART PEACE
Embracing Life's Adversities
Adolfo Quezada

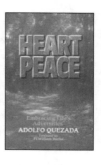

"This is one of the most authentic books I have ever read on the gut-wrenching conditions that cause or lead to human suffering. . . . His book is a gift, allowing others to be the beneficiaries of his spiritual journey" **—Antoinette Bosco**
No. RP 117/04 ISBN 1-878718-52-5 **$9.95**

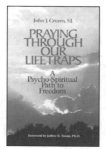

PRAYING THROUGH OUR LIFETRAPS
A Psycho-Spiritual Path to Freedom
John J. Cecero, S.J.

"John Cecero's unique book can be read not only as a primer on lifetrap therapy and practice but as a spiritual guide to finding God in all things."
—Joseph R. Novello, M.D.
No. RP 164/04 ISBN 1-878718-70-3 **$9.95**

GRACE NOTES
Embracing the Joy of Christ in a Broken World
Lorraine V. Murray

". . . will help you to see what we should be able to see naturally, but for some reason it takes grace to recognize grace! Her book is well named."

—Fr. Richard Rohr, O.F.M.

No. RP 154/04 ISBN 1-878718-69-X **$9.95**

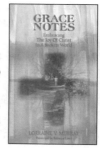

OTHER BOOKS OF INTEREST

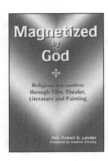

MAGNETIZED BY GOD
Religious Encounters through Film, Theater, Literature and Art
Robert E. Lauder

". . . In Magnetized by God [the author] suggests that in great art God may be reaching out to us and through our experience of great art we may be able to encounter God."
—*Liv Ulmann*

No. RP 132/04 ISBN 1-878718-92-4   **$8.95**

THE EDGE OF GREATNESS
Empowering Meditations for Life
Joni Woelfel

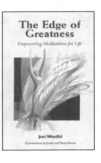

"Here is a woman whose courageous and passionate spirit has enabled her to step over the edge of greatness. She knows how to walk on water, because she has kept her eyes on the One who created the waters. Read this book and be blessed." —*Macrina Wiederkehr, OSB*

No. RP 134/04 ISBN 1-878718-93-2   **$9.95**

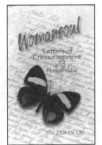

WOMANSOUL
Letters of Encouragement and Possibility
Pat Duffy, OP

". . . challenges without threatening or judging and encourages readers to step bravely toward the shining truth that each is a treasure cherished by God. Armed with that reality a woman can begin to reach into the infinity of her own soul. —*Liz O'Connor, Editor*

No. RP 152/04 ISBN 1-878718-68-1   **$7.95**

FEASTS OF LIFE
Recipes from Nana's Wooden Spoon
Father Jim Vlaun

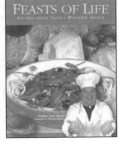

"Filled with wonderful stories and even better-sounding recipes . . . The dishes are easy to make and don't require fancy ingredients. Includes a prayer for grace, a cooking equivalents table and a cross-referenced index. —*Crux of the News*

No. RP 168/04 ISBN 1-878718-76-2   **$12.95**

Additional Titles Published by Resurrection Press, a Catholic Book Publishing Imprint

A Rachel Rosary *Larry Kupferman*	$4.50
A Season in the South *Marci Alborghetti*	$10.95
Blessings All Around *Dolores Leckey*	$8.95
Catholic Is Wonderful *Mitch Finley*	$4.95
Discernment *Chris Aridas*	$8.95
Edge of Greatness *Joni Woelfel*	$9.95
Feasts of Life *Jim Vlaun*	$12.95
Grace Notes *Lorraine Murray*	$9.95
Healing through the Mass *Robert DeGrandis, SSJ*	$9.95
Healing Your Grief *Ruthann Williams, OP*	$7.95
Heart Peace *Adolfo Quezada*	$9.95
How Shall We Celebrate? *Lorraine Murray*	$6.95
How Shall We Pray? *James Gaffney*	$5.95
The Joy of Being an Altar Server *Joseph Champlin*	$5.95
The Joy of Being a Bereavement Minister *Nancy Stout*	$5.95
The Joy of Being a Catechist *Gloria Durka*	$4.95
The Joy of Being a Eucharistic Minister *Mitch Finley*	$5.95
The Joy of Being a Lector *Mitch Finley*	$5.95
The Joy of Being an Usher *Gretchen Hailer, RSHM*	$5.95
The Joy of Marriage Preparation *McDonough/Marinelli*	$5.95
The Joy of Music Ministry *J.M. Talbot*	$6.95
The Joy of Praying the Psalms *Nancy de Flon*	$5.95
The Joy of Praying the Rosary *James McNamara*	$5.95
The Joy of Preaching *Rod Damico*	$6.95
The Joy of Teaching *Joanmarie Smith*	$5.95
The Joy of Worshiping Together *Rod Damico*	$5.95
Lessons for Living from the 23rd Psalm *Victor Parachin*	$6.95
Lights in the Darkness *Ave Clark, O.P.*	$8.95
Loving Yourself for God's Sake *Adolfo Quezada*	$5.95
Magnetized by God *Robert E. Lauder*	$8.95
Meditations for Survivors of Suicide *Joni Woelfel*	$8.95
Mercy Flows *Rod Damico*	$9.95
Mother Teresa *Eugene Palumbo, S.D.B.*	$5.95
Mourning Sickness *Keith Smith*	$8.95
Our Grounds for Hope *Fulton J. Sheen*	$7.95
Personally Speaking *Jim Lisante*	$8.95
Power of One *Jim Lisante*	$9.95
Praying the Lord's Prayer with Mary *Muto/vanKaam*	$8.95
5-Minute Miracles *Linda Schubert*	$4.95
Sabbath Moments *Adolfo Quezada*	$6.95
Season of New Beginnings *Mitch Finley*	$4.95
Season of Promises *Mitch Finley*	$4.95
Sometimes I Haven't Got a Prayer *Mary Sherry*	$8.95
St. Katharine Drexel *Daniel McSheffery*	$12.95
What He Did for Love *Francis X. Gaeta*	$5.95
Woman Soul *Pat Duffy, OP*	$7.95
You Are My Beloved *Mitch Finley*	$10.95

For a free catalog call 1-800-892-6657
www.catholicbookpublishing.com